Nurses' Aids Series

EAR, NOSE AND THROAT NURSING

NURSES' AIDS SERIES

ANAESTHETICS FOR NURSES

ANATOMY AND PHYSIOLOGY FOR NURSES

ARITHMETIC IN NURSING

EAR, NOSE AND THROAT NURSING

MEDICAL NURSING

MICROBIOLOGY FOR NURSES

OBSTETRIC AND GYNAECOLOGICAL NURSING

ORTHOPAEDICS FOR NURSES

PAEDIATRIC NURSING

PERSONAL AND COMMUNITY HEALTH

PHARMACOLOGY FOR NURSES

PRACTICAL NURSING

PRACTICAL PROCEDURES

PSYCHIATRIC NURSING

PSYCHOLOGY FOR NURSES

SURGICAL NURSING

THEATRE TECHNIQUE

TROPICAL HYGIENE AND NURSING

Nurses' Aids Series

Ear, nose and throat nursing

FIFTH EDITION

BY
Susanna Marshall, S.R.N., S.C.M., D.N.(LONDON), R.N.T.

Formerly Principal Tutor at the Hitchin School of Nursing, Sister Tutor at the Radcliffe Infirmary, Oxford, the Royal Infirmary, Doncaster and St Bartholomew's Hospital, London

AND

Zena E. Oxlade, S.R.N., R.N.T.

Principal Nursing Officer (Teaching) at the West Suffolk Hospitals

FOREWORD BY

J. McG. Jackson, F.R.C.S., D.L.O.

Consultant E.N.T. Surgeon, Ipswich and Bury St Edmunds Hospitals

BAILLIÈRE TINDALL · LONDON

© 1972 BAILLIÈRE TINDALL
7 & 8 Henrietta Street, London WC2E 8QE

*A division of Crowell Collier and Macmillan Publishers **Ltd***

First edition, May 1953
Second edition, January 1958
Third edition, September 1962
Fourth edition, July 1967
   Reprinted July 1969
Fifth edition, 1972
   Reprinted November 1974

ISBN 0 7020 0433 2 Limp edition

ISBN 0 7020 0440 5 Case edition

Published in the United States of America by
The Williams & Wilkins Company, Baltimore

Made and printed in Great Britain by
William Clowes & Sons, Limited
London, Colchester and Beccles

Foreword

IT is nearly twenty years since the first edition of this book was published. Each new edition has proved more popular than its predecessor, and its circulation has become world-wide with foreign language translations. This popularity should be maintained with the Fifth Edition.

Otolaryngology has seen changes in the incidence of diseases over the years. The techniques of diagnosis and surgery have become more sophisticated with the universal use of the operating microscopes for ear, nose and laryngeal examination and treatment. New drugs have been discovered so that specific remedies are available thus reducing the necessity for surgery in some cases but also permitting surgery when previously it had been impossible. In the field of radiotherapy new techniques mean that cures can be expected where before only palliation was available. These changes mean that nurses must have a greater knowledge of allied subjects.

This book which the authors have brought right up-to-date now draws upon the best teaching and practice in current use at several centres. As experienced tutors, Miss Marshall and Miss Oxlade have struck a balance between the practical and theoretical aspects of nursing so that the nurse understands the disease of the patient and its treatment. No book can ever replace the tutor or instil the principles of good nursing, but this book points the student in the right direction and gives details of procedures which may be unfamiliar to those nurses new to the speciality.

Wherever Ear, Nose and Throat Surgery is practised this book will be essential reading for all nurses whether undergraduate or graduate and will form a part of the teaching curriculum.

JAMES McG. JACKSON

Preface

THE aim of this book is to present the subject of Ear, Nose and Throat Nursing clearly and practically so that the nurse may learn what is normal, understand abnormal conditions and cooperate in the aims of the medical profession to restore normal function. In this way, combining knowledge and skill with a constant concern for the physical and mental comfort of the patient, a satisfying branch of nursing may be undertaken.

This new edition attempts to bring the book completely up-to-date and detailed revision has been made throughout the text. New sections have been added on Noise and on Secretory Otitis Media, and the Radiotherapy chapter has been rewritten. Particular attention has been paid to the revision and improvement of the diagrams for this edition.

I have enjoyed the cooperation of Miss Zena Oxlade, Principal Nursing Officer (Teaching), West Suffolk Hospitals. She has been closely involved with the revision of the whole book, and I am delighted to welcome her as co-author. I also gratefully acknowledge the assistance of several specialist contributors. Mr James McG. Jackson has written the Foreword, the section on Secretory Otitis Media, and has given advice on many points. Dr D. G. Bratherton of Addenbrooke's Hospital, Cambridge, has rewritten the chapter on Radiotherapy, and Mr W. Wiseman, Senior Medical Laboratory Technician in charge of microbiology at the West Suffolk General Hospital has assisted with the updating of the material on infection and its treatment by antibiotics. Dr R. A. Yorston has kindly given permission for the use of his illustrations which appear as Figures 8, 10, 11, 28 and 29.

May 1972 SUSANNA MARSHALL

Contents

Foreword   v

Preface   vii

SECTION I. INTRODUCTORY

1. General Anatomy, Physiology and Personal Hygiene of the Ear, Nose and Throat   1
2. Hygiene in the Ear, Nose and Throat Unit   10
3. The Out-Patients' Department   15
4. Nursing Techniques   26
5. Some Important Drugs used in Ear, Nose and Throat Nursing   39
6. Radiotherapy   48

SECTION II. THE NOSE AND ACCESSORY SINUSES

7. Anatomy of the Nose and Paranasal Sinuses   53
8. Diseases of the Nose   64
9. Diseases of the Paranasal Sinuses   82
10. Surgical Operations on the Nose and Paranasal Sinuses   87

Section III. The Pharynx

11	Anatomy of the Pharynx	104
12	Diseases of the Throat	108
13	Tonsillectomy and Adenoidectomy	127

Section IV. The Larynx, Trachea and Œsophagus

14	Anatomy of the Larynx. Voice Production. Swallowing	137
15	Diseases of the Larynx	144
16	Operations on the Larynx and Pharynx	160
17	The Inhalation or Ingestion of Foreign Bodies—Endoscopy	174
18	Diseases of the Œsophagus	181

Section V. The Ear

19	Anatomy of the Ear	187
20	Physiology of the Ear. Deafness	199
21	Diseases of the External Ear	206
22	Diseases of the Middle Ear	212
23	Diseases of the Inner Ear	225
24	Operations on the Ear	233
	Appendix—Glossary of Instruments	239
	Index	257

Section I: Introductory

1

General anatomy, physiology and personal hygiene of the ear, nose and throat

Introduction

Patients suffering from diseases of the ear, nose and throat are best nursed in a special section of a general hospital. The department, commonly spoken of as "Ear, Nose and Throat", is often labelled "Department of Oto-laryngology" or given an even more elaborate title, and as some of the work is carried out in semi-darkness, I have found that nurses are apt to look upon work in such a department as shrouded in mystery. The principles of nursing the patient are, however, exactly the same as in other branches of medicine and surgery. A knowledge of the positions and interrelations of the structures involved will considerably help the nurse to "unravel the mystery". More detailed anatomy will be given in the special sections of this book, but a brief outline here will perhaps be helpful in enabling her to deal intelligently with her patients.

The nose, the accessory air sinuses and the throat are all parts of a complicated cavity situated in the face and this cavity has passages leading to it from the orbits, the ears and the trachea and œsophagus. Examination of Fig. 1 will show the connection between these parts.

Mucous Membrane—A Protective Mechanism

The continuous layer of mucous membrane which lines the ear, nose and throat is so vitally important to the health of the individual that more must be said of it. It lines the nasal cavities, with the exception of the

Fig. 1.—Sagittal Section of the Nose, Mouth, Pharynx and Larynx.

vestibules and is firmly blended with the periosteum and perichondrium of their walls. It lines the lacrimal duct and is continuous with the conjunctiva. It extends throughout the pharynx, to the middle ear via the pharyngotympanic (*Eustachian*) tube, throughout the air sinuses, the larynx and lower air passages, and also, although we are not concerned with this part of the body at the moment, it lines the alimentary canal.

Over the conchæ and septum of the nose, the mucous membrane is very thick and vascular, but it is thin on the floor of the nose, in the meatuses and in the air sinuses. In the pharynx and larynx it is more loosely attached, with a considerable amount of submucous tissue, but below the level of the vocal cords it is once more closely adherent to the underlying structures. Owing to the thickness of the mucous membrane, the nasal cavities are narrower and the conchæ more prominent than they appear in the skeleton. In inflammatory conditions, the membrane is liable to be very swollen from effusion. With a cold in the nose this is commonly sufficient to block the nasal passages completely. A much more dangerous state can arise with "œdema of the glottis"; the larynx may be occluded and asphyxia result. Œdema of the glottis (especially in the sub-glottic space and loose tissue around the arytenoids)

Fig. 2. — Ciliated Mucous Membrane from the Lining of the Air Passages.

occurs also with non-inflammatory affections such as giant urticaria and serum sickness.

The mucous membrane is well supplied with blood vessels, and in most parts contains many *mucous glands*, some "goblet cell" in type and some tubulo-alveolar, which open on its surface.

The mucus secreted by these glands keeps the membrane moist. As illustrated in Fig. 2, the epithelium forming the surface layer of cells in the respiratory tract is mainly columnar and ciliated. These *cilia* are microscopic projections from the free surface of the epithelial cell, and, in health, are in constant motion. They act in sections, moving forward quickly and back slowly, from eight to twelve times a second. With the strong forward movement, the cilia brush along the mucus, with which is entangled dust and bacteria. In the nose, the mucus is propelled toward the pharynx; in the bronchial tree the direction is toward the glottis. The hairs in the nostrils filter the larger particles of foreign matter from the inspired air, and the cilia complete this important cleansing function. The cilia may continue to beat strongly in the presence of infection and pus, and are commonly regenerated with the epithelium following damage to the membrane. They are slowed down with cooling and over-heating but recover when the normal temperature returns. However, drying and smoking are fatal to them. In chronic inflammation, such as that of the paranasal sinuses, the epithelium becomes so damaged that the cilia disappear. This interferes with the normal self-cleansing function, and operations have often to be performed to allow the pus which accumulates to escape.

Breathing Habits

Upon the integrity of the mucous membrane depends a great deal of man's resistance to infection, and to preserve it is the aim of preventive measures in ear, nose and throat work. A most important factor in health is correct breathing. When "out of breath" after strenuous exercise one may take in supplementary air through the mouth, but in quiet breathing the tidal air should pass freely in and out of the nose. It is sometimes necessary to close the mouth of a sleeping infant so that it shall learn to breathe correctly. Mouth breathing begins a vicious circle. Air which is inspired through the nose is drawn through the hairs inside the vestibule. It is then warmed and moistened as it passes over the mucous surfaces. Air inhaled through the mouth lacks this filtration, warmth and moisture, and the lining of the pharynx on which the cold air strikes deteriorates in the attempt to react to such unfavourable conditions. A degree of inflammation is set up causing enlargement of the adenoids. This in turn obstructs the nasal passages so that breathing through them is impossible and the child perforce becomes an habitual mouth breather.

The Use of Handkerchiefs

As early in life as possible, a child should be taught to use a handkerchief properly. Very often the sole instruction given is by a slightly older brother or sister who holds the handkerchief, nips the infant's nose and says firmly, "Now, blow!" This most admirable effort at education needs to be further supplemented by parent or nurse. The correct method of blowing the nose is to compress each nostril alternately and blow down the other. To blow forcibly down both at once while the nostrils are closed is liable to send infectious material into the middle ear via the Eustachian tube.

Each child should be provided with his own handkerchief and supervised lest it be used for such purposes as shoe polisher, duster, face towel or flannel! Should there be much nasal discharge, as in a head cold, paper handkerchiefs should be used by old as well as young, care being taken to ensure that the soiled ones are disposed of efficiently.

Constant use of a handkerchief that is harsh either by reason of its texture or because of dried nasal discharge will cause soreness of the upper lip or painful fissures around the vestibule. When linen or cotton handkerchiefs are used during respiratory infection, they should be disinfected before being washed and boiled.

Chloros or Dettol 1 in 80 is a satisfactory disinfectant if the handkerchiefs are immersed in this for eight hours.

Respiratory Infection

Most respiratory, and many other diseases begin with the *common cold*, spread by droplet infection—that is, micro-organisms from one person's nose and throat are projected in a fine spray of saliva to the mucous membrane of a second person. There, should the second person be susceptible, they will penetrate and multiply. The common cold is the greatest cause that exists of loss of time from occupation, and therefore much research has been devoted to discovering its cause and toward preventing its spread.

Since the use of the electron microscope it has been found that several strains of virus may cause the common cold. Experiments upon healthy individuals living in strict isolation have proved that these viruses are responsible for the early symptoms—that is, the nasal irritation, the dry sensation (generally in the nasopharynx), the sneezing, followed in a few hours by profuse discharge of watery mucus, and general malaise. After a simple virus infection there is a gradual return to normal in three to seven days. In ordinary life the individual is exposed to other pathogenic bacteria, such as *Neisseria catarrhalis*, streptococcus, staphylococcus, pneumococcus, and *Hæmophilus influenzæ*. It is the increase of these organisms that appears to be responsible for the more advanced symptoms of a cold—the purulent nasal discharge, the sore throat, and the sinusitis.

There are several known predisposing factors. In over-heated rooms, the air tends to dry the film of mucus covering the nasal and oral cavities. The cilia, which move the mucus, and with it, the dust and germs, then become less active. The dried mucus forms crusts inside the nostrils, and there, especially if the nose is picked with the finger-nail, is a potential site for the entrance of pathogenic bacteria. Sometimes anatomical abnormalities, such as deviation of the septum, so alter air currents inside the nose that they impinge on one spot in the posterior nares and so cause drying.

Defence Against Infection

Experiments at the Common Cold Research Unit have disproved many long-standing preconceptions as to the causes of colds, such as exposure to cold or long standing in wet garments. However, clothing appears to be a factor in relation to respiratory infections, especially in children. Underclothing should be light in weight and loosely woven to enmesh air which is a poor conductor of heat. As few garments should be worn as are consistent with comfort. In cold weather warm coats and strong shoes should be provided for outdoor wear, and children must not be expected to be too "hardy". A quick reaction of the skin to changes in temperature is something to be encouraged, but it must not be presumed to be automatic in all individuals or too early in life.

The general resistance to infection also depends on an *adequate, well-balanced diet.* Regular, wholesome meals are essential to health, and extra vitamins, especially A, C and D, are protective against respiratory infections. Ascorbic acid, cod-liver oil and malt, halibut-liver oil or Adexolin capsules, or similar preparations containing vitamins are justifiably much used during the winter months, but they do not take the place of a sufficiency of food. The habit of omitting breakfast and having a "snack lunch" predisposes to infections of the respiratory tract. It leads to fatigue—another factor which lowers resistance.

Adequate hours of sleep in a ventilated room, with warm but not heavy bedclothes, are essential to health.

It is important to avoid overcrowding and to maintain good ventilation in all situations of work, leisure, sleep and meals. During outbreaks of respiratory infectious diseases, the avoidance of crowded public places, such as cinemas and large department stores should be strongly recommended.

Attempts have been made, with some success, to create an immunity to colds by the injection of vaccines. For some specific diseases—diphtheria, whooping cough, poliomyelitis—vaccines are widely used, particularly in early life.

The Spread of Respiratory Infection

During quiet breathing the range of droplet spread is usually 2 to 3 metres, but droplets may be carried 18 metres or more by currents of air. The spread is much increased by the sneezing and coughing, with which so many infectious diseases commence. It is during the onset of the disease therefore, that persons are most highly infectious.

There is a variety of pathogenic organisms which tend to multiply in the mucous membrane of the nose and throat. Many individuals harbour organisms to which they themselves are immune, but which may produce clinical attacks in others. Such individuals are known as "carriers". Diseases commonly transmitted by carriers are the various manifestations of infection by the hæmolytic streptococcus, diphtheria caused by the corynaebacterium diphtheriae, and cerebrospinal meningitis caused by the meningococcus. Recently the carriage of *Staphylococcus aureus* (often resistant to antibiotics) in the nostrils has assumed great importance in hospital and carriers are excluded from contact with wounds. It must be borne in mind that hæmolytic streptococci are responsible for many diseases including scarlet fever, tonsillitis, cervical adenitis, sinusitis, otitis media, mastoiditis, skin sepsis, impetigo, wound suppuration, cellulitis, erysipelas, puerperal fever and septicæmia. All patients with such diseases should be nursed by isolation technique, preferably in a single room or in a cubicle. If possible, all nurses attending them should be immune.

2

Hygiene in the ear, nose and throat unit

Building Construction

An ideal Ear, Nose and Throat unit should be self-contained, consisting of an Out-Patients' Department, an operating theatre equipped with its own anæsthetic and instrument rooms, and wards for in-patients. There may be a separate dressing room and a post-operative intensive care unit. The spacing of the beds in the wards is an important consideration. The incidence of carriers is greatly increased by overcrowding, and cross-infection becomes inevitable in a ward where beds are too close together. The distance between the bed centres should be not less than 3.6 m or, if beds face each other, there should be 5.2 m between the two heads. Wards are best sub-divided by glazed screens 2.35 metres high, with a 15 cm clearance of the floor for cleansing, into some single-bedded cubicles (particularly in the section for young children) and some four-bedded wards. This limits the spread of infection, and ensures more privacy and quiet for the patients who can at the same time be under observation by the nursing staff through the glass partitions. The wards should be light and airy, and the ventilation as free as possible. In some units, a Plenum ventilation system is installed, providing positive pressure in treatment rooms, negative in the sluice room. If the beds are placed parallel to the long axis of the ward, the patients do not directly face the light. Often, balconies or verandahs are provided, and patients should be encouraged to use these both winter and summer. Even if balconies are not available, almost open-air conditions can be achieved in the ward if one or more walls are largely windows.

Cross-Infection and its Prevention

Ward dust contains millions of bacteria. These are mostly harmless, but pathogenic organisms are usually present. In the Ear, Nose and Throat ward of one hospital the floor sweepings were estimated to contain 100 million hæmolytic streptococci. Staphylococci, diphtheria bacilli, pneumococci, tubercle bacilli have also been found. The bacteria emanate from bedclothes, personal clothes and dried droplets. Blankets of patients with upper respiratory infections harbour a great many germs which are scattered into the air at every bedmaking or movement of the blankets. Dust which is raised settles again to contaminate furniture, bedclothes, patient's clothing, or is inhaled by persons in the ward.

Should pathogenic organisms be present in sufficient quantities, and should they fall on susceptible tissues, infection will thus be spread.

Ward Hygiene

In order to reduce dust-borne infection, ward cleaning should be done by vacuum and damp dusting. No dry dusting should be allowed.

Wool blankets are now largely replaced by cotton ones of the terry-towelling or cellular weave. These are easily washed and sterilized. The accepted minimum is a clean set for every patient, but the objective in an Ear, Nose and Throat ward, is to change the blankets every three days, or even every day. Where wool blankets are still in use, they should be sewn inside cotton covers—particularly for theatre use.

Soiled linen should never be counted, sluiced or washed in the ward, but put into bags at the bedside;

the bags are then sealed and taken to the laundry. Linen used by patients suffering from respiratory infection should be put at the bedside into alginate bags sewn with material which dissolves during washing.

Nursing Principles

The nursing staff must apply aseptic principles to their work. These will safeguard the patients (all of whom may not be infectious), the nurses, and the visitors.

Each patient should have separate thermometer, towels, soap, flannels, comb, hair brush, toothbrush and a supply of paper tissues. Fresh disposable tray cloths should be supplied at each meal. The patient's temperature should not be taken in the mouth if the patient is unable to breathe through the nose.

In many Ear, Nose and Throat wards, if bedpans and urinals are not disposable, they are sterilized after each use, and the feeding utensils are boiled after each meal. Thus, the necessity of keeping them marked for each patient is obviated. Feeding utensils after use should be washed in water of over 75°C with detergent and should be kept in cupboards, or otherwise protected from dust.

The hands of the nursing staff should be thoroughly washed with soap and water *before* preparing or giving meals, before examining a patient, before dressing a wound, and *after* attending to a patient's oral or nasal toilet, dealing with excreta, soiled linen or pathological specimens, cleaning, dusting or guarding a sneeze. After washing, the hands should be well dried and a cream such as Hibitane rubbed in.

Linen roller towels should not be used, but an adequate number of clean dry towels should be provided. Destructible paper towels are an advantage. A supply of paper handkerchiefs should be issued to each patient, and a paper bag attached to the locker. Each handkerchief should be used once only and then be placed in the bag, which can be burnt with its contents.

Efficient face masks should be worn by the staff when carrying out aseptic procedures. The mask should cover nose, mouth and chin and is usually disposable, being made of special paper. It should be discarded after use and should never be kept in the nurses' pocket. A plentiful supply should be kept in the ward in a covered container near the hand-washing basin.

The admission of patients is the duty of the medical officer who will endeavour to avoid admitting those who are suffering from, or incubating an infectious disease. In the ward, however, it is often the sister or nurse who is in a position to detect the earliest signs of an incubating infection. The early transfer of a patient into a single-bedded room or discharge to his home may check an epidemic.

Should an outbreak of an infectious disease occur in a ward, all patients showing signs of the infection should be barrier nursed or sent to an isolation unit. Antiserum is given to those post-operative patients who have not had the infection. All those who are particularly susceptible to the infection should be kept under close observation.

During the incubation period of the disease, all patients should be kept in bed and examined for early signs and symptoms. The admission of new patients should cease until there is no danger of further spread of the infection. For example, if diphtheria occurs, no new patients should be admitted; if whooping cough, no new patients under three years should be admitted. The admission of children for tonsillectomy should also be suspended when severe epidemics, e.g. of poliomyelitis, measles, scarlet fever, are prevalent in the neighbourhood. The operation is not performed on children who have not been immunized against poliomyelitis.

The noses, throats, wounds or discharges should be examined bacteriologically, and the patients should not be regarded as free from infection until at least two successive negative swabs, at an interval of not less than three days, have been obtained. All members of the ward staff who show any sign or symptom of infection by hæmolytic streptococci—whether it is sore throat, severe cold, skin sepsis (especially of fingers) or other manifestation—should be taken off duty until they have ceased to be carriers. However willing a nurse may be to sacrifice herself to her duty, she must remember that when she is not well she may be a serious danger to her patients, and should therefore not delay in reporting early signs of infection. This is particularly important in an Ear, Nose and Throat Department where many of the patients are children whose immunity is not fully developed. The majority of patients moreover, are already suffering from an inflammation of the mucous membrane and are therefore susceptible to infections other than those causing the original disease. Should a chronic carrier of infection—that is, one who harbours the germ long after all signs of the disease have disappeared—be found among the staff, he or she must be excluded from the ward.

3

The out-patients' department

The Out-Patients' Department is a very important part of an Ear, Nose and Throat Unit. Many patients receive treatment here and do not need admission to the ward. Those who are admitted to the ward are first examined in the Out-Patients' Department, and some minor operative procedures are performed there.

The Department should have an ample waiting hall for patients, so that over-crowding is avoided. It should have adequate ventilation and heating, artificial ventilation being installed in some cases. There should be a number of consulting and examination rooms or cubicles, a surgery or small theatre, and one or two small "recovery" rooms. In addition, an office for secretarial work should be provided.

The Examination Room

Furniture.—The room in which the patient is examined must frequently be darkened by blinds. Therefore a good artificial light is required. A standard lamp of the angled type is used for inspecting the patient, the light being reflected from a head mirror worn by the surgeon. Alternatively, a head lamp may be used. The patient sits in a chair of which there are several types. A swivel chair may be used. The standard lamp on a movable stand is placed on the left side of the patient's chair. The surgeon, wearing the head mirror on his forehead, sits opposite the patient. At the surgeon's right hand there should be a table, on which the instruments required for various examinations are laid. Beneath the table there should be a soiled-dressing bin with a lid. This may conveniently be of the type whose lid is operated by a foot-lever. Paper bags are provided for lining the bin. The bags are burnt after use and the dressing bins are emptied and disinfected daily. A supply of stationery, including request forms for pathological investigation and X-ray examination, and instructions for home treatments, should be put in a convenient place; also a supply of paper handkerchiefs and of packets of absorbent paper ("Medical Wipes").

Examination Table.—On the table, the instruments should be laid out as follows:

1. The surgeon's head mirror, or head lamp.
2. Cotton wool, of the finest absorbent quality.
3. Jobson-Horne ring probes and aural orange sticks (the wool is wound round these, for the purpose of absorbing moisture from cavities).
4. Clean dressing towel, for drying instruments.
5. Receiver for soiled instruments.
6. Spirit lamp and box of matches. (These are for warming mirrors and specula; some surgeons prefer to use boiling water.)
7. Bowl of Hibitane 75 per cent. in spirit for disinfecting mirrors which cannot be boiled.

The instruments required for examination:

8. Nasal specula.
9. Aural specula.
10. Tongue depressors.
11. Laryngeal and post-nasal mirrors.
12. Metal probes or orange sticks.
13. Aural forceps.
14. Nasal forceps.
15. Tuning fork.
16. Eustachian catheters.
17. Politzer bag.
18. Auscultation tube, the vulcanite end pieces of which, after use, are placed in Hibitane.

19. Siegl's speculum.
20. Rogers or De Vilbiss spray.

Cleaning of Instruments.—After use, instruments are scrubbed with a brush under running cold water and, in some departments, in Hibitane (chlorhexidine) solution, after which they must be rinsed. If the hospital has a central supply of sterile articles, they are returned to that department. Otherwise, those which are boilable (not mirrors or vulcanite articles) are then boiled for 5 minutes in water to which bicarbonate of soda may have been added in the proportion of 5 ml to 1 litre of water. Mirrors must never be boiled, unless marked "boilable". They may be dipped quickly into boiling water and then immersed in Hibitane 75 per cent. in spirit for at least 20 minutes in order to disinfect them and are then rinsed in plain water and dried.

Wooden spatulæ and orange sticks are broken after use, and thrown into the bin for soiled dressings.

At the end of the day, all instruments should be dried and carefully examined, those needing repair being placed on one side and the matter reported to the sister in charge. New nurses should be warned that the angle of a post-nasal mirror is intentional, and that they should not, in their zeal, attempt to straighten it!

Drugs Used on Examination Table

1. Cocaine hydrochloride 10 per cent. solution.
2. Adrenaline 1–1000 solution.
3. Anæsthetic lozenges, e.g. amethocaine.
4. Cocaine paste 25 per cent.
5. Ephedrine 1 per cent.
6. Penotrane (Hydrargaphen) 0.4 per cent. in absorbent starch base powder in an insufflator.
7. Antibiotic preparations.
8. Hydrocortisone and neomycin ointment.

Examination of the Patient

Ideally, the examiner and all attendants should be masked.

Inspection of the face as a whole may have bearing upon nasal conditions.

Mouth breathing is revealed by the shape of the mouth which is narrowed and held open. Blockage of the nasal passage, such as occurs with enlarged adenoids, leads to constant sniffing on the part of the child, and this causes suction on the roof of the mouth which results in arching of the palate, a narrow jaw, and overlapping of the incisor teeth. The facial appearance is generally termed "adenoid facies".

Fig. 3.—The Adenoid Facies.

Collapse or expansion of the alæ nasi, widening of the bridge of the nose, fulness over the accessory sinuses, or soreness of the vestibule and upper lip, are frequent indications of nasal infection.

When a child is to be examined, a few minutes spent in gaining his or her confidence may often avoid struggles. If the nurse is required to hold the child she should realize that she can neither gain his co-operation nor restrain his head movements by grasping his hands—the correct method of holding him is shown in Fig. 4.

FIG. 4.—HOLDING A CHILD FOR A THROAT EXAMINATION.

An adult's head is usually steadied between the hands of the nurse, who stands behind him.

Examination of the Nose

It is usually the nurse's duty to dress the probes immediately before they are required. If prepared long in advance, the wool may become loose. Cotton wool, of a long-fibred absorbent quality is used. It is especially teased for the purpose, and may be provided in sterilized cartons. If a wooden carrier is moistened first, the wool will adhere more firmly. A wisp is placed on the end of the probe so that part projects in a loose tuft; the remainder is twisted firmly round the probe with the fingers. The nurse should test it to ensure that the wool will not become dislodged during use.

Taking a Swab of the Anterior Nares

No treatment should be applied to the area for at least six hours beforehand.

The patient is seated facing a good light. A sterile swab is taken from a sterile test tube, passed into one nostril for 25 mm to 50 mm and rubbed gently but

FIG. 5.—POST-NASAL SWAB IN POSITION.

firmly round the nasal fossa. If a membrane is present the swab should be placed on it. The swab is then withdrawn and replaced in the sterile tube, which must be suitably labelled and sent to the laboratory without delay.

Sometimes swabs may be required from both nostrils and should be marked "Left" and "Right".

Taking a Post-nasal Swab

This procedure may be carried out on persons suspected of carrying the meningococcus of cerebrospinal meningitis. The oral route is used, and a swab mounted on a bent wire is employed.

A good light is essential. The tongue should be depressed by a spatula so that the swab can be directed to the required position without touching the sensitive uvula (Fig. 5) and without becoming contaminated with saliva.

Bacteria commonly found in the nose and throat are: Streptococcus viridans, *Neisseria catarrhalis*, and various micrococci.

Infective organisms are: hæmolytic streptococci, pneumococci, influenzal bacilli, corynebacterium diphtheriae, staphylococci and viruses. *Candida albicans* causing "thrush" (ref. page 119) may follow the use of broad-spectrum antibiotics.

Aural discharge in acute otitis media may contain influenzal bacilli, pneumococci or streptococci and staphylococci; in chronic otitis media it frequently contains staphylococci, *Bacillus proteus*, and *Pseudomonas pyocyanea*. Occasionally, there are certain species of fungus—notably the aspergillus species.

For some examinations, the nose may require spraying or preliminary packing in order to anæsthetize it.

Before examination of the ear, the external ear may need syringing to clear it of wax. These nursing techniques are also carried out in the ward and are described in Chapter 4 (page 33).

Examination of the Ear

The external aspect of the ear gives little or no information as to its internal condition. Radiography may show this to a certain extent. A mastoid abscess may cause bulging behind the auricle and push it forward.

To test hearing, tuning forks of varying pitch are required. These help to indicate degrees of deafness and whether the cause lies in the middle or the inner ear. Deafness is discussed in Chapter 20.

Examination of the Tympanum

The normal eardrum is a grey transparent membrane closing the inner end of the external auditory canal and lying at an angle with it in a double slant. It is easily seen with an auriscope. It is a tense membrane (hence the name "drum") and described on page 190.

Through the drum can be seen the malleus of the middle ear, and below this a cone of light (reflected light, see Fig. 37, page 190) spreads downwards. After syringing the ear the healthy drum often appears pink. With infection it becomes first red and later opaque and thickened. Swelling of the meatus may obstruct the view of the drum.

Before examination, the ear should be inspected. Any wax, pus or debris should be removed and the meatus dried. Syringing is the best method, but must be used only on instruction.

FIG. 6.—HOLDING THE AURICLE FOR EXAMINATION OF THE EAR.

Examination with Head Mirror and Speculum

The patient should be sitting if possible. Several sizes of speculum should be available. The examiner holds the warmed speculum between the thumb and forefinger and inserts it into the meatus which is straightened by drawing the auricle up and back with the middle and ring fingers. For an infant, the auricle is drawn down and back, as the bone is not fully developed. The nurse shines a light into the head mirror. A mirror is unnecessary with an electric auriscope which gives a magnified image.

In some ear diseases the drum is indrawn or bound by adhesions. To test its mobility, *Siegl's speculum* is used. This instrument consists of a rubber bulb and tube, to which is attached an end-piece into which is screwed a lens. This lens is warmed over a spirit lamp, to prevent condensation of moisture upon it.

An aural speculum is fitted to the end-piece and inserted into the ear. If the bulb is compressed when inserting the speculum, relaxation of the bulb, by producing a negative pressure in the meatus, will tend to draw the eardrum outwards. By varying the air pressure, an otherwise invisible perforation may be detected.

The condition of the pharyngotympanic tube, which may be obstructed or may contain mucus, is investigated by inflation of the middle ear.

1. **Valsalva's Method.**—The patient should close the mouth, nip his nostrils and try to blow forcibly. If the tubes are patent, air is forced up them and the patient will hear a click as air enters the middle ear. The examiner may confirm this by watching through a speculum for movement of the tympanum, or listening via an auscultation tube.

2. **Politzer's Method.**—This method is used most often on children. The child holds a sip of water in the mouth. The nozzle of the Politzer's bag is inserted into one nostril and then both are closed so that no air can escape. The child is told to swallow and at the moment of swallowing, the bag is compressed and air is driven into the middle ear. During swallowing the orifices of

the pharyngotympanic tubes are opened; the soft palate rises and shuts off the nasopharynx from the parts below.

3. Inflation by Eustachian Catheter.—In this method one tube only is inflated at a time. The catheter (page 243), metal, usually silver, has a curved beak to fit into the orifice of the pharyngotympanic tube, and at the other end, a ring on the same side as the curve, to indicate its position when hidden. The catheter is passed along the floor of the nose until it touches the posterior pharyngeal wall. It is then turned point outwards and gently withdrawn until it passes into the pharyngotympanic tube. An air bag is then attached to the catheter, and air driven gently up the tube. An auscultation tube may be attached to a stethoscope connecting the ear of the patient with that of the surgeon who can then hear the air blowing into the middle ear if the pharyngotympanic tube is patent. Bubbling sounds indicate the presence of pus; a whistling sound, a perforation of the drum.

The auscultation tube (page 245) is fitted at each end with a vulcanite end-piece—one black and one white. The surgeon usually chooses the white end-piece to place in his own ear.

The nurse should be very careful over the cleaning and drying of the catheters. Being made of soft metal, they bend easily and may become dented with rough handling. After cleaning, air should be blown through with the Politzer bag to make sure that they are patent.

Before examining the ear of a very young child, a general anæsthetic is given; a Eustachian catheter is passed via the nose by the surgeon, and the tube is inflated whilst the surgeon examines the ear with an auriscope.

Examination of the Throat

The larynx cannot normally be seen by direct vision;

by passing an illuminated tube-spatula, the soft tissues of the throat can be so displaced that the interior of the larynx and its surrounding parts can be seen. This is called "direct laryngoscopy". "Indirect laryngoscopy" is the examination by means of a mirror and will be described here. The patient may be recumbent or sitting, with the head extended. The method of holding a child is shown in Fig. 4. The nurse stands or sits behind the patient so that he does not back away from the surgeon. A good light is essential and a hand lamp or torch may be needed.

If examining with a torch only, a tongue depressor should be placed over the centre of the tongue, pushing it gently down. It should not be placed far back, as this may make the patient retch. If a laryngeal mirror is used, the tongue is held forward in a paper tissue. The mirror is warmed in the water or in the flame of the spirit lamp. This prevents "misting" by the patient's breath.

The examiner should test the heat of the mirror on his own hand or cheek before putting it in the patient's mouth. During the examination, the doctor asks the patient to say "ee-ee" as this causes approximation of the vocal cords.

4

Nursing techniques

Cleansing the Nostrils

Once a child has learnt to blow its nose, mechanical cleansing of the nostrils is unnecessary in health. Occasionally crusts may be present inside the nose when there is local disease. These may require softening with liquid paraffin; the nostrils are subsequently swabbed with sodium bicarbonate solution, 10 ml to 600 ml of water, or with normal saline.

The swabs are well moistened and held in nasal forceps, or wire wool-carriers may be used. Before treatments on the nose the patient should blow it.

Insertion of Nasal Drops

These are ordered chiefly when vasoconstriction is required, ephedrine $\frac{1}{2}$ per cent. in normal saline being the common solution or Tuamine Sulphate $\frac{1}{2}$ per cent. A glass dropper with a rounded end and a thin rubber bulb is convenient—if the dropper is incorporated in the stopper of the bottle containing the fluid care should be taken that it is replaced immediately without contamination. The fluid should be slightly warmed before insertion. The patient may sit with the head forward while the drops are being inserted and should tilt the chin up, but not too far; otherwise the drops run down the floor of the nose into the pharynx and are swallowed. Usually however, the patient is placed on his back, with the head over the edge of the bed (see Fig. 7) and turned from one side to the other, as each nostril is being treated. The patient should be told to breathe through the mouth. While drops are being instilled

NURSING TECHNIQUES

into one nostril, the other is compressed with a finger.

To supplement the use of drops, pledgets of cotton wool dipped in the lotion may be inserted under the middle conchæ and left for a short time.

FIG. 7.—POSITION OF PATIENT FOR INSERTION OF NASAL DROPS.

Spraying the Nose.—The apparatus used is a nasal or throat spray, the glass part of which must be sterilized. After filling the spray with lotion and expelling the air, the patient's head should be held forward over a receiver and the nozzle inserted into the nostril. By gently compressing the rubber bulb, the fluid is injected with very slight force and is allowed to flow down the other nostril. It is important that the patient should breathe through the mouth whilst this is being done.

Oily fluids and antiseptic solutions are seldom

used for nasal drops and sprays. Oil may be inspired into the lungs and cause pneumonia. Antiseptics, water, and strong salt solutions have been found to interfere with ciliary action. The isotonic saline solution of ephedrine recommended above has no harmful effect on the ciliary movement and flow of mucus.

Packing the Nose

The nose may require packing:

(a) To arrest obstinate hæmorrhage, when the procedure is usually performed by a doctor using gauze impregnated with bismuth and iodoform paste. A cocaine spray is applied before packing.

(b) To anæsthetize it before operation or examination, when the responsibility generally rests with the nursing staff. The manner in which the nose is packed may make all the difference between a comparatively painless operation and one associated with discomfort and delay. Ribbon gauze, 13 mm wide, with a selvedge, is the material used for plugging, and two pieces, each 1 m long are required. Each nostril should be packed with one piece only. If more are used, there is danger that one piece may be left behind when the packing is removed. This would set up irritation, infection and possibly ulceration.

Requirements:

1. Sterile gallipot containing 8 ml of cocaine 10 per cent. solution in which the two lengths of ribbon gauze are soaked. (Cocaine is a dangerous drug; the amount must be prescribed by a doctor, and checked by a competent person. Some surgeons may order a larger amount of a weaker solution, e.g. 30 ml of 5 per cent. cocaine.)
2. Gauze plugging.
3. Nasal forceps.

NURSING TECHNIQUES

4. Dissecting forceps.
5. Dressed wool carriers.
6. Scissors.
7. Sterile wool swabs.
8. Receiver.

Method.—The patient is seated facing a good light. The nurse puts on her mask and prepares the dressing trolley with the above apparatus. She then washes her hands thoroughly and dries them on a clean towel and returns to the patient. The patient should be given the

FIG. 8.—ANTERIOR NASAL PACK.

receiver and told to spit out any fluid which may find its way into his throat. She picks up the end of the plugging, which should be soaked in but not dripping with the cocaine solution, with the nasal forceps. While supporting the other end of the plugging with dissecting forceps, she carries the first end into the nostril straight along the floor of the nose to the back of the nasal cavity. The nostril is packed firmly and gently, passing the plugging under the inferior turbinate and then under the middle turbinate bone.

The other nostril is then packed in the same way. The nurse must beware lest the packing be pushed into the nasopharynx and swallowed.

To obtain the full effect of the cocaine, the above procedure should be carried out 15 minutes before the operation.

Another method of anæsthetizing the nose is to smear 10 or 25 per cent. cocaine paste over the mucous membrane lining the nasal cavity. The paste is commonly issued in screw-cap tubes and is applied by means of wool carriers. The carriers are inserted into each nostril and held in position for 20 minutes by a piece of adhesive strapping fixed below them, the ends reaching the bridge of the nose.

Suction Displacement Therapy

Conditions of chronic maxillary sinusitis present difficulties of treatment, due to the anatomical structure of the maxilla. It is possible, however, to admit fluid to the sinus, by applying suction to the nose when the patient's head is in such a position that the opening of the sinus is below the level of the fluid. The result is that air is drawn from the cavity, and the fluid replaces it.

Method.—The patient lies on his back with a pillow under his shoulders, his neck straight and his head well back (as in Fig. 7). A Dakin or Proetz syringe is required, and about 5 ml of warm lotion—usually ½ per cent. ephedrine or tuamine sulphate in normal saline. The patient is told to breathe through his mouth and to continue saying "Kick, kick, kick". This raises his soft palate and shuts off his nasal cavities. Whilst one nostril is being treated, the other is closed with a finger. The end of the syringe is kept inside the nose, the rubber bulb is squeezed while the patient says "Kick" and released when he stops to breathe. This is done two or three times. The patient may then rest and sit up. He

Steam Inhalations

The periodic inhalation of steam is a treatment much used in the relief of sinusitis and other respiratory infections. There are on the market specially shaped earthenware inhalers with separate mouthpieces of glass or earthenware (useful only for throat and chest treatment) but for most purposes in nose and throat work, a 1-litre jug with a wide top is preferable. An astringent drug is usually vaporized and inhaled in the steam. Some that are commonly prescribed are:

(*a*) Pine and menthol mixture, 5 ml to 600 ml of water.

(*b*) Compound tincture of benzoin (friars' balsam), 5 ml to 600 ml of water.

(*c*) Menthol crystals, 1 or 2 to 600 ml of water.

In order to avoid scalding the patient's throat, and to obtain the maximum effect of the vapour, the water for the inhalation should be at a temperature of 71°C (160°F). This is obtained by using approximately 150 ml of cold water and adding 450 ml of boiling water.

Requirements.—A tray containing:

1. The inhalant in an airtight bottle.
2. Teaspoon, or measure.
3. Lotion thermometer.
4. Jug containing 600 ml of water at 71°C (160°F), covered with a wool or flannel bag, and standing in a bowl.
5. Towel to twist round the top of the jug to prevent the steam escaping into the room.

Method.—The patient is first made to blow the nose. If she is up, she should sit at a table on which the inhalation tray is placed. If in bed, she is best sitting with her back well supported by pillows. A patient who is unable to sit up may be treated in the lateral position. No very ill or very young patient should be left during an inhalation. The tray is brought to the patient's side, and the prescribed amount of the inhalant is floated on the water, so that none of the vapour is lost. The jug in the bowl is given to the patient and placed so that she can bend her head and inhale the steam without effort.

If the patient is sitting in bed a pillow may be placed over her knees. Sometimes it is considered an advantage to cover the patient's head and the jug with a bath towel. Certainly it may help the patient to concentrate on the treatment in process but the nurse cannot then observe her patient so easily. A better method is to fold a towel in tubular form round the rim of the jug. The patient can then hold the upper edge of the towel to fit round the nose and mouth and thus avoid steaming the face and head. The patient is told to breathe in and out through the mouth for about 10 minutes. In most conditions for which inhalation is prescribed, the nasal passages are closed by swollen mucous membrane, so that breathing through them is impossible. Often this treatment opens up the passages.

When the inhalation is finished, the patient's face is dried, her hair is combed, and she is covered with the bedclothes. Patients must be warned not to expose themselves to cold air for at least half an hour, and preferably for 2 hours after inhalation.

If a Nelson's or a Maw's inhaler is used, the water is allowed up to the lower border of the air inlet only. This precaution is taken partly to prevent spilling and partly so that the steam is driven freely from the surface of the fluid. The mouthpiece is fitted into the inhaler in such a way that the air-inlet will point away from the patient who holds the mouthpiece, which may be covered with a layer of gauze, between the lips. After use, the mouthpiece is washed and then boiled for 5 minutes. The fluid used for an inhalation is poured away and the jug or inhaler is cleaned and dried. Should tincture of benzoin have been used, stains are easily removed with a swab moistened in methylated spirit.

Spraying the Throat

It is sometimes necessary to spray the throat with a local anæsthetic before a posterior rhinoscopy, endoscopy (especially bronchoscopy), or before dissection of tonsils. The solution used is 10 per cent. cocaine, to which may be added 0.06 ml of adrenaline 1-1000. 1 ml of the cocaine solution is usually sufficient, and the maximum anæsthetic effect occurs about 15 minutes after application.

Method.—The patient is first given a mouth wash. The solution is put into a Rogers's spray and the tongue is sprayed. This is then held down whilst the pharynx and epiglottis are sprayed.

An alternative, and more generally used, method of anæsthetizing the throat is to give the patient a tablet of benzocaine or amethocaine to suck 20 minutes before the examination.

Syringing the Ear

This procedure is dangerous in unskilled hands because of the risk of perforating the ear drum. A nurse should not syringe an ear without instructions from a doctor. If the purpose is to dislodge a foreign body, he himself will carry out the procedure, but for other treatments, the responsibility is usually passed on to the nurse. Should it be required to remove an accumulation of wax in the ear, drops of warm sodium bicarbonate, or other solution should be inserted before syringing. Sodium bicarbonate saponifies the wax so that it is washed out easily. Some aural surgeons favour a mixture for the drops, of:

    Sodium bicarbonate   ..   4 parts
    Glycerin .. .. .. 10 parts
    made up to 100 parts with normal saline.

Others prefer:

    Sodium bicarbonate .. .. 25 parts
    Glycerin .. .. .. 10 parts
    made up to 100 parts with normal saline.

Others again use warm oil, for example, olive oil, or its substitute arachis oil, instead of sodium bicarbonate. The oil softens the wax, which then, however, tends to be driven nearer the drum.

The drops should be inserted into the external meatus several hours before syringing, preferably on the previous evening.

Requirements:

1. *Either:* A metal ear syringe with a removable nozzle; *or:* A Higginson's syringe with a straight Eustachian catheter.

2. Head light, or head mirror to reflect light from a lamp.

3. Lotion in a litre measure:
    (*a*) Normal saline solution;
or (*b*) Salt and sodium bicarbonate solution (5 ml of each dissolved in 1 litre water).

4. Lotion thermometer.
5. Aural forceps.
6. Dissecting forceps.
7. Gallipot of fine wool swabs.
8. Receiver for the lotion—this may be a kidney bowl, or be specially shaped. It may be of vulcanite so that any pus or wax in the returned fluid shows up clearly against the black of the dish.

NURSING TECHNIQUES

9. Paper bag for soiled swabs.
10. Receiver for soiled instruments.
11. Mackintosh cape.
12. Dressing towel.

The temperature of the lotion is very important. If it is much above or below the body temperature the patient will suffer from giddiness or may faint. The lotion should be at a temperature of 38°C (100°F) in the jug, when commencing the irrigation.

If a metal syringe is being used, the nurse should ensure that it is working smoothly. A Higginson's syringe is never boiled, but the aural nozzle or the Eustachian catheter is sterilized by boiling. When there is any wound, or discharge of the ear, strict aseptic technique is necessary.

Method (for one nurse).—The patient sits with the ear to be treated towards the operator, and holds the

FIG. 9.—SYRINGING THE EAR, SHOWING METHOD OF HOLDING SYRINGE.

receiver close against the cheek under the ear. The nurse fixes the mackintosh cape and towel over the patient's shoulders. She then puts on her head lamp, or, if this is not available, the head mirror, and arranges

Fig. 10.—TECHNIQUE OF SYRINGING. THE TIP OF THE SYRINGE IS JUST IN THE MEATUS AND THE JET OF WATER IS DIRECTED ON TO THE POSTERIOR CANAL WALL.

Fig. 11.—REMOVAL OF A FOREIGN BODY.

NURSING TECHNIQUES

the lamp so that the light can be reflected from the mirror. She then washes and dries her hands, takes the syringe and attaches the nozzle. The syringe is filled with lotion and the air expelled. With one hand she draws the pinna upwards and slightly backwards to straighten the external meatus, and with the other hand she holds the syringe and directs the lotion first along the roof of the canal, then along its floor. When the irrigation is finished, the ear is gently dried with cotton wool, the wool being firmly held so that it projects in a loose tuft beyond the point of the forceps.

Irrigation of the Maxillary Antrum

In some cases of chronic maxillary sinusitis, the surgeon will make an intranasal antrostomy into the antrum considerably lower than the natural ostium. After the operation he may order daily irrigation of the antrum which is the nurses' duty to carry out.

Requirements:

1. Higginson's syringe, with an adaptor to fit the cannula.
2. Antrum cannula.
3. Jug containing 1 litre of normal saline solution.
4. Lotion thermometer.
5. Kidney bowl.
6. Mackintosh cape.
7. Dressing towel.
8. Paper bag for soiled swabs.

Method.—The nurse inserts the cannula by passing it gently straight into the nostril with the curved beak of the cannula pointing outwards. (The ring at the other end of the cannula is on the side of the curve.)

When the opening into the antrum is felt, the cannula is twisted so that it points downward and outward. The patient bends the head forward and holds the kidney dish under the chin to catch the wash-out lotion. The nurse then attaches the Higginson's syringe, from which all air has been expelled. During the irrigation she uses her free hand to hold the patient's head steady. (See Fig. 13.)

Fig. 12.—Passing the Antrum Cannula.

Fig. 13.—Irrigation of Antrum.

This procedure must not be confused with the antral puncture when no permanent artificial opening is made. For this treatment see p. 91.

5

Some important drugs used in ear, nose and throat nursing

Local Anæsthetics

Local anæsthetics may be used to produce complete insensibility to pain in a particular area of the body. One of the drugs most frequently used for this purpose is *cocaine*. Cocaine has little action on the unbroken skin, but if applied to mucous membrane it produces complete local anæsthesia, so that small operations can be performed without the patients feeling them. For ear, nose and throat work the drug is commonly used in strengths 10 to 25 per cent. aqueous solution of cocaine hydrochloride. Not only does its power of penetrating mucous surfaces make it an efficient anæsthetic, but the vasoconstriction that it induces is of great value, particularly in the nose. The consequent shrinkage of the mucous membrane improves visibility and access to the passages and assists sinus drainage. The action of the drug is increased and prolonged by the addition of 0.06 ml of adrenaline solution 1–1000 to each 1.3 ml of cocaine used.

In place of cocaine solution which is sprayed on mucous surfaces, cocaine paste is frequently used. This is a compound of cocaine (usually 25 per cent.) and suprarenal extract in a mixture of liquid paraffin and petroleum jelly. The great advantages of this paste are that it keeps indefinitely and that absorption of cocaine is minimal.

Owing to its toxicity and its tendency to produce addiction, cocaine is listed as a Dangerous Drug and can be obtained only on the signed prescription of a doctor. It must be kept in a locked cupboard which is used only for such poisons.

The toxic effects are pallor, sweating, shallow breathing and a fall in blood pressure. The pulse at first quickens, then becomes slow and feeble. There may be nausea and vomiting, and should cerebral irritation occur there are convulsions. Death may follow from heart failure or from asphyxia. Cocaine is specially dangerous to children under six years of age, and for all ages it is too toxic for injection into the tissues. The first-aid treatment for cocaine reaction is to lower the patient's head, loosen the clothing round the neck, open the nearby window and give oxygen. If the patient can swallow, he may be given water, sal volatile or brandy. The most up-to-date remedy is intravenous Pentothal.

For local anæsthesia produced by subcutaneous injection cocaine has been largely superseded by substitutes such as procaine and amethocaine. These are less effective as surface anæsthetics but are less toxic and do not produce addiction. They are not subject to the regulations of the Dangerous Drugs Act but the dose must be adequately checked at the time of administration. A so-called idiosyncrasy to a local anæsthetic is probably due to accidental absorption into the blood stream either during injection or through a wound in the mucous membrane to which the anæsthetic is applied. To avoid the possibility of cerebral disturbances, all patients due to have a local anæsthetic of cocaine should be given a barbiturate, such as 100 mg of Nembutal, the night before. The adrenaline that some surgeons add to the cocaine solution is used in order to diminish local absorption of cocaine.

Cocaine may cause excitement in some patients, and if used in the treatment of an out-patient, he should be allowed to rest for at least half an hour before leaving hospital.

SOME IMPORTANT DRUGS

After the throat has been cocainized for direct endoscopy (see page 174), the cough reflex will be absent for some time, and special precautions must be taken that the patient does not inhale fluid or food. Nothing is given by mouth for two hours, then the patient is given a glass of water to sip slowly.

Drugs to Combat Infection

The discovery this century of drugs which will harm invading organisms more than living tissue has revolutionized treatment of infection. The two main groups of these drugs—sulphonamides and antibiotics—are bacteriostatic or bacteriocidal according to their concentration. Sulphonamides act by competing for the raw materials necessary for the existence of the organisms. The result is that, since the bacteria are prevented from growing and multiplying, the natural defences of the body can deal with them. When the influence of the drug is withdrawn, the remaining organisms resume growth and multiplication. The aim is to keep the drug in contact with the infected tissue until the infection is overcome. Antibiotics act more directly. Some will block an essential enzyme but Penicillin for instance acts on the cell wall of the bacterium so that this is imperfect and the organism finally ruptures under osmotic pressure. Other act directly on bacterial cell contents. The drugs are rapidly absorbed and eliminated (although there are newer long-acting compounds) or diffuse rapidly from any site of local application; therefore repeated administration during this period is necessary.

The essential value of these drugs is in the treatment of acute infection. They are relatively ineffective in chronic infections, more particularly in chronic types of disease, possibly because these are often of an allergic rather than an infective nature. In all cases, resistant strains of organisms occur, and laboratory tests must be made to discover the agents to which the organisms are sensitive.

Chemotherapy—Sulphonamides

Systemic treatment by a sulpha drug is frequently adopted for serious streptococcal infections particularly where there is danger of meningitis, but its use is uncommon for pharyngitis of average severity, since in the first place, neither the duration nor the severity of the disease is markedly lessened by its use, and, in the second, the possible dangers inherent in the use of these drugs are greater than those of the infection. If sulpha therapy is considered advisable, the preparations usually chosen are *sulphadiazine* or *sulphamezathine*, the latter being the less toxic. Both are rapidly absorbed and eliminated, therefore large initial doses are ordered, followed by smaller maintenance doses which must be given both night and day. A usual prescription is 2 to 4 grammes to be given at once, then 1.5 grammes 4-hourly until symptoms subside. A sodium bicarbonate mixture is frequently ordered with each dose. For children, the amount of sulpha is calculated by their weight, giving 0.1 gramme per pound per day. The amount of the drug given must be recorded. Sulphonamides (usually Sulphadiazine) are the primary treatment of choice in meningitis because of the ease with which they cross into the cerebrospinal fluid.

During the administration of a sulpha drug a large amount of fluid should be taken by the patient in order to prevent crystallization in the kidneys. (This complication, however, is extremely rare with sulphamezathine.) The amount of fluid intake and output should be recorded, and the urine tested daily. Should hæmaturia or anuria occur, the drug must be stopped at once, but the alkaline mixture should be continued. The doctor must be informed immediately.

SOME IMPORTANT DRUGS

Another rare danger of sulpha therapy is agranulocytosis. Nearly every patient gets some reduction of leucocytes, which usually appears after 6 days. Should an early reduction occur the drug is discontinued. The same applies if fever has not abated in 48 hours.

Sulpha drugs may produce toxic effects in a person sensitized by previous administration, which is another argument against the routine use of the drugs in mild infections. These toxic effects include high fever, cyanosis, skin rashes, a red sore throat, headache, loss of appetite, nausea and vomiting.

Antibiotics

These are drugs prepared from living moulds or other bacteria, and constitute the most recent group of drugs used against infection. Their action depends upon the inhibitory effect exerted by one organism on another—"antibiosis". During the last few years, many such drugs have been used because of their activity against different organisms. The most important of these are:

Penicillin, effective against Gram positive organisms and certain spirochætes
Streptomycin, effective against Gram negative organisms and certain acid-fast bacilli

Ampicillin
  (Penbritin)
Chloramphenicol
  (Chloromycetin)
Tetracycline
  (Achromycin)
Oxytetracycline
  (Terramycin)
Chlortetracycline
  (Aureomycin)

These are called "broad-spectrum" antibiotics, being effective against many organisms, including some large viruses. Since they tend to sterilize the small intestine, large doses of vitamin B are usually given with them.

Erythromycin
Neomycin
Nystatin — This antibiotic is specific for fungal organisms.

Methicillin Sodium (Celbenin)
Cloxacillin Sodium (Orbenin) — Used for resistant staphylococci.

Penicillin.—In a virulent infection for which sulphonamides are ineffective and which is sensitive to penicillin this is the antibiotic most often used, partly because it is cheap and readily available, and partly because, apart from the hypersensitivity which some people develop towards it, it is relatively non-toxic. Being a large-moleculed substance it does not diffuse as readily as sulphonamides. It is given by injection deep into the muscle. One scheme is to give a high dose of crystalline penicillin, for example 500,000 units or even 1–2,000,000 units, followed by a similar dose in 12 hours. The theory is that the first dose produces a high level in the blood and is excreted in 4 hours; the second dose produces another high level when any remaining organisms are ready to divide. This method removes the need for frequent needle-pricks. Other methods involve the six or eight-hourly doses of 300,000 to 1,000,000 units of one of the more more slowly absorbed preparations over several days. Capsules and tablets for oral use are now widely prescribed, but the absorption of penicillin by this route is uncertain and the effects on the mucosa of the mouth and colon may require counteraction by doses of vitamin B. This is because non-pathogenic bacteria normally living in the colon and helping in the absorption of vitamin B are destroyed by oral antibiotics. An extra supply of the vitamin is therefore needed.

Penicillin must be kept cold when in solution,

although the crystals in a dry state are fairly stable. In the presence of water, the drug rapidly loses its effect and contamination with organisms from the hand can destroy its effect. Therefore, the nurse should use a dry sterile syringe and the usual aseptic procedure for giving the injection. At the same time, in order to avoid developing hypersensitivity to the drug, she should keep all traces of penicillin solution off her own hands. Any excess solution drawn into the syringe should be returned to the phial before withdrawing the needle—it should not be squirted into the air. She should wash her hands carefully after cleaning the syringe. Rubber gloves may be worn as a protection.

Streptomycin.—This antibiotic may be used to combat certain organisms that are insensitive to penicillin, notably the tubercle bacillus. It has not been used to a great extent in Ear, Nose and Throat work except for tuberculous conditions. Streptomycin has an effect on both the vestibular and auditory functions of the inner ear, and deafness has several times been attributed to its use. The usual dosage of streptomycin is 0.5 grammes twice daily until 15 grammes have been given. The drug is then discontinued except in tuberculosis.

Chlortetracycline (Aureomycin).—This drug differs from the preceding antibiotics in that it is usually given by mouth. It is particularly useful against *Staphylococcus aureus*. Although it is not absorbed so quickly into the blood as is penicillin it disappears more slowly. The usual dosage is 0.5 to 1 gramme every four hours until 12 to 14 grammes have been taken.

Chloramphenicol (Chloromycetin).—This drug was originally derived from a mould but is now prepared synthetically. Like aureomycin, it is given by mouth, usually in capsular form, though it can be absorbed rectally. Unlike aureomycin, it contains a nitrobenzine factor in its composition, which can cause a severe form of anæmia, and therefore it should be prescribed with caution. It is recommended that the use of chloramphenicol should be reserved for the diseases for which it is specifically valuable—whooping cough and infections shown to be sensitive to it in laboratory tests.

Oxytetracycline (Terramycin).—This is still another antibiotic, useful when organisms are penicillin-resistant. It can be given by mouth—2 grammes daily for fourteen days, and is also prepared as a 1 per cent. ointment or in powder form for insufflation.

Neomycin.—This is an antibiotic too toxic to give by mouth or injection but useful as a local application in ears because it acts on *Pseudomonas pyocyanea*. It is an ointment, often combined with cortisone.

Orbenin and **Celbenin** are given by injection.

Polymyxin.—This is the name given to a group of five polypeptide antibiotics produced from *Bacillus polymyxa* and named A to E. Polymyxin B is the best of the series and is effective against many organisms including *Pseudomonas pyocyanea* and *Escherichia coli*. It is used for local or general treatment and prepared as 1 per cent. drops, 2 per cent. ointment or for parenteral injection. The usual course is 250,000 units intramuscularly every 4 hours for 5 days.

For severe infections of the ear, nose or throat, it is customary to prescribe immediately a sulphonamide and penicillin. Laboratory tests are made, if necessary, to discover whether the organisms responsible for the infection are sensitive or resistant to the drugs in use. Guidance can then be given as to the type of drug and the dosage which would be most helpful.

There is need for co-operation between the ward and laboratory to control hospital infection. Genetic changes in bacteria can cause significant alterations in the infection pattern.

Cytotoxic Agents

Certain malignant conditions of the head and neck

may be treated by drugs known as cytotoxic agents. These drugs interfere with the cell metabolism, and malignant cells are particularly sensitive to their effects. Considerable destruction and regression of tumour tissue has been achieved by their use. They are highly toxic and dosage should be carefully controlled. Frequent blood counts are needed as a leucocytosis will occur. Nurses should be aware of the side effects and watch for and report these. Side effects are skin rashes, urticaria, nausea, vomiting and diarrhoea. Severe gingivitis is sometimes seen. Frequent mouth care is necessary for the patient's comfort.

Methotrexate.—This is an antimetabolite. Absorption is rapid and the drug is excreted unchanged within 12 hours. Oral tablets of 2.5 mg are used. For parenteral use sodium methotrexate is prepared in 5 mg and 50 mg vials; it must be reconstituted with water. In treating tumours of the tongue and glands of neck it can be given by continuous intra-arterial infusion. This method ensures that the tumour receives the maximum dose of the drug. Depending on the site of the tumour, a small-bore cannula can be inserted in the external carotid artery, the superior thyroid or lingual arteries. Fluorescein or methylene blue may be injected to ascertain that the cannula is in the correct position. A dose of 50 mg in 24 hours is usually aimed at. In the whole course about 750 mg are given. A specially adapted infusion apparatus is required to allow the reservoir to be at least 10 feet above the patient to overcome the arterial pressure. Sufficient tubing should be used to allow the patient freedom of movement as the infusion may continue many days. Toxic effects may be lessened by giving folic acid systemically.

Mustines.—Nitrogen mustard can be given by simple arterial injection. Phenylalamine may be used also. As soon as the leucocyte count returns to normal, oral therapy may be substituted.

6
Radiotherapy

Radiotherapy is the treatment of disease with X-rays or gamma rays. These have a selective action on malignant cells and cause damage to the nucleus preventing cell division. There is also some temporary damage to normal cells which shows itself as the radiation reaction, but if the dose of X-rays is carefully regulated, this reaction settles down quickly and a cure results.

It is important to keep the irradiated area small in order to produce as little disturbance to the patient as possible. In the tongue, this can be done by implanting radioactive needles or seeds directly into the tumour. If, however, the growth has spread more extensively or has involved the glands of the neck it is preferable to use X-rays administered externally.

For many years radium was the only radioactive material available and when first produced it was extremely expensive and was guarded with care by the nursing staff. After the discovery of the atom bomb nuclear reactors were developed and materials such as radioactive gold, iridium, cobalt and caesium became available. These can be produced in larger quantities and are gradually replacing radium. The rays they produce are not so penetrating and simplify storage and protection problems.

It is important for the nurse to realize what dangers are associated with radioactivity, but at the same time to keep these in perspective. The more actively dividing tissues are most sensitive to radiation and large doses can affect the blood and ovaries causing anaemia and sterility. These doses are never likely to be reached with the small amount of radium used in needle implantation treatments and even the patient will not be affected in this way.

Staff who are responsible for the safety of radioactive materials are specially designated and have routine checks of radiation received. This ensures that they do not receive more than the tolerance dose which is laid down by the authorities. The nurse who looks after the occasional case is not likely to reach this dose and is not usually tested in this way.

Implantation Techniques

Radium

In this method needles containing radium are inserted in a planned pattern to produce uniform dosage throughout the tumour. The needles are made of platino-iridium and contain from 0.5 to 3 mg of radium inside an inner platinum cell. They are threaded on silk to enable them to be removed.

A general anæsthetic is given and the position of the needles checked by an X-ray film. These are left in place for a week and are examined twice a day to ensure that none is working loose. The threads are usually secured firmly to the cheek by strapping and should not be disturbed.

A chart showing the number and type of needles is kept in the notes and a special sign showing the presence of radioactivity is displayed at the foot of the bed. During this time visitors may be allowed, but they should not sit close to the bed and should be discouraged from lengthy visits.

The nursing treatment whilst the needles are in place is chiefly directed towards maintaining the patient's nutrition and keeping the mouth as clean as possible. A special liquid diet can be provided, but it is often more convenient and certainly more palatable to put the normal diet through a liquidizer to break down solid particles. After each meal the mouth should be irrigated with normal saline to wash away food particles from the needles and their threads.

At the end of the calculated time, the needles are removed usually by the medical staff and returned to the safe. If they are placed far back in the tongue an anæsthetic may be required. They are carefully counted, and as an extra precaution the patient is surveyed with a portable radiation monitor to be quite sure that all radium has been removed.

Radioactive Gold

This has a short half-life of 2.8 days and has therefore become largely inactive after 2 to 3 weeks. It is used in the form of small "seeds", 3 mm long, which can be implanted into the tissues and left there permanently. These seeds are put in with a special gun carrying a cartridge of 15 seeds. They do not interfere with movements of the tongue and little special nursing care is required. The patient needs only a short stay in hospital, usually 2 or 3 days.

Radioactive Iridium

In this technique, nylon tubes are inserted into the tongue and their position checked by an X-ray film before they are loaded with the radioactive iridium wire. This cuts down the exposure to medical and nursing staff in the Theatre and X-ray departments.

X-ray Therapy

When the tumour is no longer localized to a small area, external X-ray therapy is used. There is no difference in the action of the gamma rays from radium and the X-rays produced by electrical machines. It is merely a question of how deep into the tissues they penetrate, and this depends on the voltage at which the X-rays are generated.

Deep X-rays produced at 250,000 volts have been used for many years, but they are now being replaced by X-rays from linear accelerators at 4 to 6 million volts or by the rays from radioactive cobalt. Both these have the advantage that they cause little skin reaction and can easily penetrate bone and cartilage which may be involved with tumour. The less penetrating deep X-rays tended to be absorbed by these tissues which were therefore overdosed causing pain and necrosis. The development of these newer radiotherapy machines has greatly reduced the discomfort of X-ray therapy.

It is still necessary to treat as small an area as possible and often a special jig or mask is constructed for each individual patient, so that several beams of X-rays be accurately directed to the tumour site. Treatment is given over 4 to 5 weeks often as an outpatient and the daily progress of tumour and reaction is observed.

An optimistic and encouraging attitude is essential during this extended treatment, especially when the inevitable discomfort of the reaction begins. Radiation to the mouth and neck reduces the amount of saliva and mucus and causes a dry mouth and loss of taste.

Two-hourly fluid or soft feeds should be advised and the patient should also be encouraged to drink as much as possible of bland fluids. He will not want to eat very hot or seasoned foods. Moreover, 14 g of mucilage containing 500 mg of aspirin given half an hour before meals makes swallowing very much easier.

The skin reaction is not usually a problem, but the soreness and redness of the erythema can be reduced by a spray containing hydrocortisone. Skin marks used in the planning of the treatment should not be washed off without medical permission. When large areas of the trunk or abdomen are treated the patient may have a general reaction with headache and nausea. This is not a problem where only the neck area is treated. If the patient feels sick or nauseated in any way he should be treated with Largactil or Fentazin.

Hyperbaric Oxygen Therapy

It is now known that large tumour masses have areas which are poorly supplied with blood vessels where the cells are lacking in oxygen. This makes them difficult to kill with radiation and the centre of the tumour may require more dose than the normal tissues can stand to kill the anoxic cells.

The problem is to get more oxygen to the blood stream and from this to the anoxic cells. This can be achieved by increasing the pressure at which oxygen is breathed. A special hyperbaric chamber of perspex is used in which the patient lies during treatment. He wears special antistatic clothing to minimize the risk of sparking and subsequent fire. The pressure is increased gradually over the first 15 minutes until 3 atmospheres is reached and this is maintained for a further 15 minutes to allow oxygen to soak through the tissues. Treatment is then given through the wall. During the whole of this time the radiographer talks to the patient through the headphones. As the pressure increases the patient is told to swallow to prevent pressure changes in the ears. Some radiotherapists perform a myringotomy before treatment and insert grommets into the ear drums to avoid pressure changes and subsequent pain. This, however, is not essential.

The oxygen method is still under trial in many centres and is not universally available. Initial results suggest that it may be very useful in tumours around the head and neck.

Section II: The Nose and Accessory Sinuses

7

Anatomy of the nose and paranasal sinuses

The nose is the first section of the respiratory passage, and extends from the roof of the mouth to the base of the skull and from the anterior to the posterior nares. It is divided into right and left nasal cavities by a septum, which is bony posteriorly but is composed of cartilage anteriorly. Air enters the nose through the nostrils (or anterior nares) and passes into the pharynx through the posterior nares.

For purposes of description the nose is divided into an external and an internal portion.

The External Nose

The external portion of the nose projects forwards from the centre of the face in a variety of shapes and sizes. The more or less pointed tip is called the *apex*, the part between the apex and the upper lip is the *base*. Where the nose joins the forehead is the *root* of the nose, and extending from the tip to the root is the *dorsum* of the nose, the portion nearest the root being called the bridge. The rounded eminence lateral to each nostril is called the wing of the nose, or the *ala nasi*.

The framework of the external nose is partly of bone and partly of cartilage. The aperture of the bony part of the external nose is, as seen in a skull, somewhat the shape of a heart upside down, being bounded by the maxillæ in the lower two-thirds and by the two nasal bones in the upper third. The nasal bones are interposed between the frontal processes of the maxillary bones.

The cartilaginous portion of the framework of the external nose consists of five major cartilages—the right and left lower nasal cartilages (forming the tip of the nose), right and left upper nasal cartilages, and the septal cartilage interposed vertically between these cartilages so as to form almost the whole of the septum of the anterior part of the nasal cavity—and several small alar cartilages which lie behind the lower nasal cartilages and above the fibro-fatty tissue of the alæ nasi. The five major cartilages may be variously fused to one another and to the bones by the continuity of the perichondrium and periosteum. The anterior-inferior portion of the septum is freely movable; it is not formed by the septal cartilage but by the septal processes of the lower nasal cartilages and by the skin. The tip of the nose can, therefore, be pulled up, down and around.

Muscles and Nerve Supply of the External Nose.—Small slips of muscle arising from the *fascia* over the nasal bones and inserted into the skin between the eyebrows, produce transverse wrinkles over the bridge of the nose; others compress or dilate the nasal apertures. All these muscles are supplied by branches of the facial nerve, whereas the skin covering the external nose is supplied by branches of the trigeminal nerve.

The Skin of the Nose.—Over the bony portion of the external nose, the skin is thin, and since it rests upon loose subcutaneous tissue containing very little fat, it is freely movable. As it approaches the tip and base of the nose, the skin becomes a little thicker, and the subcutaneous tissue is much denser, becoming fibro-fatty in nature, which means that the skin loses its mobility. It also acquires many large, sebaceous glands, the openings of which in relation to the very fine hairs are readily seen.

Blood Supply.—The external nose is supplied by a

ANATOMY OF THE NOSE

rich arterial network from several sources. Passing on to the nose near its root is a branch of the ophthalmic artery (from the internal carotid). From the side comes a small branch of the internal maxillary artery (from the external carotid). Just above and just below the ala run branches of the facial artery. These arterial

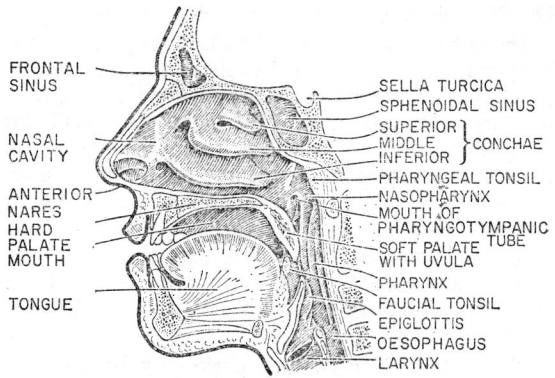

Fig. 14.—Sagittal Section of the Nose, Mouth, Pharynx and Larynx.

branches anastamose with one another and with their fellows from the opposite side. The veins draining this area end in the anterior facial and ophthalmic veins. There is some anastamosis here which may become significant should infection occur, since the ophthalmic vein drains into the cavernous sinus inside the skull.

There are lymphatic capillary networks in the skin and walls of the external nose, particularly dense at the apex, alæ and root, and which drain into the submaxillary group of lymph nodes and anastamose with the lymphatics of the mucous membrane of the nasal fossæ.

The Internal Nose

The internal nose comprises the cavity, divided by the septum into a right and left nasal fossa. The shape of the fossa, seen from in front, is of a rather long and narrow right-angled triangle, with the right angle formed by the septum and the floor of the nose, and the superior angle blunted by the roof of the fossa. The shape of the fossa in sagittal section is shown in Fig. 14.

The Anterior Nares (nostrils) are in the base of the nose. They vary a great deal in size, shape and the plane in which they lie, according to the individual and the race. Directly above each naris is the slightly expanded part of the fossa which is called the vestibule. A recess of the vestibule extends forwards into the tip of the nose. The vestibule is lined by a thin skin which is tightly adherent to the underlying cartilage and fibro-fatty tissue, and contains, in the lower part of the vestibule, coarse hairs which curve downward to guard the entrance. There are sebaceous glands related to these hairs.

The Posterior Nares.—Each posterior naris is an oval opening approximately 25 mm vertically and 10 mm transversely. It is completely bounded by bone covered with mucous membrane. Above it is the body of the sphenoid; medially is the posterior free margin of the vomer; laterally, the medial pterygoid plate of the sphenoid bone; and below, the posterior border of the horizontal portion of the palatal bone.

The Roof of the Nasal Fossa is in the form of a narrow arch, the uppermost boundary being formed by the cribriform plate of the ethmoid bone (through which pass branches of the olfactory nerve), and the posterior sloping part by the body of the sphenoid, interrupted by the rounded orifice of the sphenoidal sinus.

The Floor of the Nose is approximately horizontal

and is formed of bone—the anterior three-quarters by the palatine processes of the maxillæ, and the posterior quarter by the horizontal processes of the palatine bones. The floor of each nasal fossa is slightly concave from side to side. Its width is, to some extent, dependent on the size of the maxillary sinus.

The Nasal Septum is composed chiefly of a very thin plate of bone called the *vomer*, the perpendicular plate

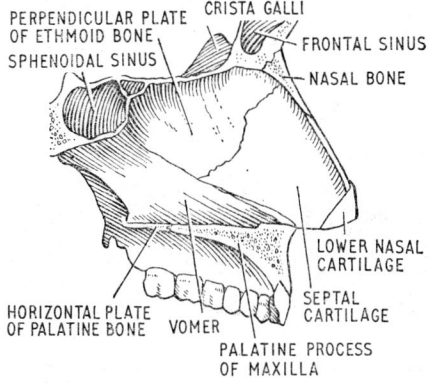

Fig. 15.—The Osseous and Cartilaginous Nasal Septum.

of the *ethmoid bone*, and the *septal cartilage*, described in relation to the external nose. Their relation to each other is shown in Fig. 15. In addition, small processes from the maxillæ, the palatine bones, the sphenoid bone, the frontal bone and the nasal bones articulate with the three main constituents of the septum named above, and so contribute slightly to the margin of the septal framework.

Above the vestibule, the *lateral wall of the nasal fossa* presents three projections with a bony foundation which run more or less horizontally and diminish in length from the lowest to the highest. These are named the inferior, middle and superior concha or turbinate respectively. The portions of the nasal fossa overlapped by these conchæ are called the inferior, middle and superior meatuses. The inferior concha is a separate bone which articulates with the maxilla, the lacrimal,

FIG. 16.—DIAGRAMMATIC SECTION OF THE NASAL CAVITY.

the ethmoid and the palatine bones. The lacrimal duct which drains the secretion of the lacrimal gland from the conjunctival sac opens into the inferior meatus. Emotion stimulates the gland. As the duct is very small it cannot cope with a highly active gland, and if there is excessive secretion, this not only drains into the nose but also overflows down the cheeks as tears. A vigorous blowing of the nose can therefore sometimes prevent crying.

The middle and superior conchæ are projections of the ethmoid bone. In the middle meatus are openings from the ethmoid air cells, the frontal sinus and the maxillary sinus. The superior meatus contains openings from the posterior ethmoid air cells. The sphenoid

ANATOMY OF THE NOSE

sinus opens into the "spheno-ethmoidal recess" which lies above and behind the superior concha.

The Lining of the Nose.—The lining of the vestibule is composed of modified skin which merges into the mucous membrane which lines the nasal fossæ proper. This nasal mucous membrane is of two kinds: olfactory and respiratory. Respiratory mucous membrane is discussed in Chapter 1. Olfactory mucous membrane is found in the upper part of the nose only—that is, over the superior concha and the adjacent part of the septum. It has a yellowish tinge, and is of stratified epithelium, containing olfactory cells which receive the stimuli which give rise to the sense of smell. Processes from the olfactory cells bundle together to form the olfactory nerves which pass through the cribriform plate of the ethmoid bone to end in the olfactory bulb.

Blood Supply.—The lining of the nasal fossæ receives its blood supply from branches of the external and internal carotid arteries. Venous plexuses form a cavernous tissue inside the nose, especially on the inferior conchæ and lower part of the septum. The blood drains into veins which more or less follow the arteries.

Lymph Supply.—Lymph vessels from the vestibule and the adjacent part of the nasal fossa, communicate with the vessels of the external nose and eventually drain into the submandibular group of the lymph nodes. There is some communication between the lymphatics of the right and left sides, particularly in the mobile septum. From the remaining part of the nasal fossa, the lymphatics run posteriorly and drain into the retropharyngeal and deep cervical glands. There is some connection between the lymphatics of the nasal fossa, through the cribriform plate of the ethmoid bone, with the subarachnoid space.

Nerve Supply.—Apart from the aforementioned olfactory nerves which are distributed to the olfactory portion of the nasal mucous membrane the nerves of the nasal fossa are branches of the trigeminal nerve. They are, for the most part, sensory fibres, but a few efferent fibres carry impulses to the glands and blood vessels in the lining of the nose.

The Accessory Nasal Sinuses

In the bones which help to form the framework of the nose are some important air spaces which com-

Fig. 17.—Diagrammatic View of the Skull to show the Positions of the Paranasal Sinuses.

1, Frontal sinuses; 2, Maxillary sinuses, opening into the middle meati; 3, Ethmoid sinuses and sphenoid sinus.

municate by relatively small openings with the nasal fossæ. There are usually two (right and left) in the frontal bone, one in each maxillary bone, and two (right and left) in the sphenoid bone, called the *frontal, maxillary* and *sphenoid sinuses* respectively, while four to eight in each lateral mass of the ethmoid bone are called the *ethmoid air cells*.

The Frontal Sinuses are usually located one each side of the midline, where the part of the frontal bone which forms the forehead bends back to form the roofs of the orbits. They are separated from each other by a thin bony septum which is usually deflected to the right or left so that the sinuses vary in size and shape. The average measurements are about 25 mm in height, 18 mm in width and 12 mm at the base, and the average capacity is 6 or 7 cm^3. Each communicates with the middle meatus of the nasal cavity by a passage called the frontonasal duct. Occasionally there are several frontal sinuses, each with a duct into the nose. Either or both frontal sinuses may be missing. Sometimes they extend deeply into the orbital portion of the frontal bone. Persons with large frontal sinuses very often, but not always, have prominent superciliary arches and to them may be ascribed (right or wrongly) great powers of concentration and intelligence, whereas the noble appearance of their foreheads is due to air, and not to brain!

The Maxillary Sinus (or "Antrum of Highmore" as it is frequently called) is situated in the body and zygomatic process of each maxilla but frequently extends into other processes of the bone. It is roughly pyramidal, its apex formed by the zygomatic process. The floor is formed by the alveolar process of the maxilla, and its lowest part is usually about 12 mm below the floor of the nasal fossa. The roof of the sinus forms the floor of the orbit. Nerves to the upper teeth run in grooves or canals through the walls of the sinus and contribute to its nerve supply. The extreme thinness of the walls of this cavity explains why tumours arising in the sinus may project upwards into the orbit, forwards on to the cheek, downwards into the mouth or inwards to the nose. Many maxillary sinuses have inward bony projections in thin ridges, especially from the floor, making pockets which are difficult to drain.

The opening into the nasal fossa is usually high in the medial wall of the sinus and leads into the middle meatus. In many instances there is an additional opening lower in the wall, but this is generally closed by mucous membrane.

The Sphenoid Sinuses lie in the body of the sphenoid bone and communicate with the nasal cavities through openings slightly above the level of the floor of the sinus. The right sphenoid sinus is divided from the left one by an extremely thin bony septum, which is rarely central, so that they are not symmetrical. Like the other sinuses, they vary very much in size, but their main development takes place after puberty. They are related above to the optic chiasma and the pituitary

FIG. 18.—DRAINAGE OF FRONTAL AND MAXILLARY SINUS (note difficulty of drainage from the latter).

gland; on each side to the internal carotid artery, the cavernous sinus and the 3rd, 4th and 5th cranial nerves; in front with the nerves and blood vessels crossing the roof of the nose to supply the nasal septum; behind, with the basilar artery and midbrain. It is interesting to note that the sphenoid sinus may be in relation to all

ANATOMY OF THE PARANASAL SINUSES

three cranial fossæ, and that the walls of the sinus may be extremely thin.

The Ethmoidal Sinuses consist of three groups of air cells; anterior, middle and posterior, which entirely occupy the lateral masses of the ethmoid bone and may extend into the neighbouring bones. The anterior and middle groups open into the middle meatus of the nose, and the posterior group into the superior meatus. The partitions between the air cells are very thin and sometimes missing—there may be an absence of bone between the anterior ethmoid cells and the lacrimal sac. Ethmoid cells which invade the roof of the orbit come into relationship with the anterior cranial fossa.

The paranasal sinuses begin to develop in fœtal life, but are only minute spaces at birth. The frontal sinuses are fairly well developed at 7 or 8 years of age, but reach their full size after puberty. The maxillary sinuses reach full size after the eruption of permanent teeth.

8

Diseases of the nose

Affections of the External Nose

Diseases of the Skin

Many who develop dermatitis or eczema of the nose suffer from the disease in other parts of the body also, and are treated in the skin wards and not in the Ear, Nose and Throat department. Some skin diseases, however, are especially associated with the nose and these will be considered here.

Acne Rosacea.—This condition is one of chronic hyperæmia of the face, particularly of the nose. There is a dilatation of blood vessels with the formation of papules and pustules with core-like centres. In later stages there is permanent enlargement of the vessels and thickening of the connective tissue.

The cause may be dietary, alcohol or hot tea being especially liable to aggravate the disease. Gastro-intestinal disturbances, emotion or the menopause may also be responsible. In all cases the main treatment is regulation of the diet. Stimulants and condiments should be avoided, also hot drinks and any articles of food found to give the patient indigestion.

Local applications with an astringent action, such as calamine or lead lotion, or a mixture of both may be used. The lotion should be repeatedly mopped over the flushed area.

Furunculosis—Boils.—A boil is the result of inflammation of a hair follicle or sebaceous gland. There is suppuration and, after a few days, the expulsion of a mass of necrotic tissue commonly known as the "core".

The causative organism is commonly *Staphylococcus aureus*, often resistant to penicillin.

The furuncles occurring in the nose generally begin at the tip. There is at first deep-seated induration developing into a round, red, throbbing prominence which becomes softer as suppuration occurs. The boil usually "points" into the vestibule and its centre appears as a yellow spot. Until the core is discharged there is much pain owing to the tightness of the skin over the nasal cartilages. There is frequently a recurrence, the site of the boil moving deeper into the nose.

With each boil there may be fewer obvious signs, but as there is less room for the skin to swell, the pain becomes more intense. The patient must be warned to resist the temptation to pick or squeeze the spot, and all nurses should understand that any septic condition of the nose, or indeed of any part of the face must be regarded seriously. There is danger of the infections spreading to the orbit and so to the cavernous sinus. A rigor, pyrexia associated with headache, and swelling of the eyelids would indicate the serious condition of sinus thrombosis. Cellulitis of the whole face sometimes accompanies nasal furunculosis.

Treatment.—The small solitary furuncle is rarely treated with antibiotics, but with recurrence one of these is given. Sometimes, local treatment of the nose will give relief—for example, frequent hot bathing, or plugging the nostril with ribbon gauze well soaked in hot normal saline or saturated boric lotion. Too strong a salt solution must be avoided as it is liable to damage the surrounding skin and mucous membrane and to leave the nose very sore. An analgesic drug, such as aspirin or an aspirin compound will probably be necessary to relieve pain and enable the patient to sleep at night. Vitamins A, B, C and D should be given to help raise his resistance against infection. Should there be pyrexia, rest in bed is indicated. When the "pointing" stage of the boil is complete, a light touch with a sharpened wooden applicator dipped in pure phenol will hasten the expulsion of the core and promote drainage, or the boil may be left to discharge itself.

To prevent recurrence, the inside of the nostril may be painted with an antiseptic solution such as Argyrol or gentian violet 1 per cent. The hairs inside the nostril should be kept closely clipped. For persistent recurrence, the use of autogenous vaccine has met with some success. A holiday and attention to the general health are advised.

Cavernous Sinus Thrombosis.—This very serious condition may be an extension of thrombosis of the angular vein, caused by furunculosis of the nose. The septic thrombus travels to the cavernous sinus via the ophthalmic vein. If there is slow occlusion of the sinus, a collateral circulation is set up. The patient is desperately ill.

Signs and Symptoms.—There are recurrent rigors, the temperature rising to 40.6°C (105°F). Nausea and vomiting frequently occur. Pain in the orbit and side of the head is acute and there is intense progressive œdema of the eyelids. The eyeball is protruded and paralysis of the eye muscles follows due to the involvement of the cranial nerves in the cavernous sinus. There may be ptosis, squint and alterations in the pupils.

Treatment.—The usual nursing for patients with intermittent pyrexia and sweating will be needed. Recovery depends largely upon the early administration of antibiotics, anticoagulants and treatment of the primary infection.

Lupus Vulgaris.—This is a chronic inflammation, now uncommon, of the skin of the nose and cheeks caused by invasion by the tubercle bacillus. Occasionally it attacks the trunk and limbs. The first sign is the appearance of one or more tiny reddish or reddish brown papules surrounded by an area of hyperæmia. When pressed by glass, the spots have an "apple jelly" appearance. They gradually enlarge, forming an irregular patch of soft nodules which often ulcerate, crust and heal with scarring. Healing occurs in one part of the affected area while spread is taking place at another. The ulcers are superficial and scars are yellowish and shrunken. The disease occurs in children and young adults. It is painless, but there is often much destruction of cartilage and bone. Occasionally the nose is destroyed, or carcinoma may develop.

Treatment.—General treatment consists of a highly nourishing diet with additional vitamins. Calciferol is given in large doses for at least a year. Ultra-violet light may be employed. Streptomycin, Para-amino salicylic acid and Isonicotinic acid may also be given.

Lupus Erythematosus.—This disease is differentiated from lupus vulgaris as there are no nodules or ulcers. There are reddish patches covered at times with an adherent scale, and there is a tendency to scarring. When on the nose, the disease often extends on to the cheeks in a butterfly-shaped patch. It is a local manifestation of what is generally a systemic disease.

Treatment.—There should be protection of the face from strong sunlight. Systemic steroids are given.

Frostbite.—Owing to its exposed position the nose is one of the first parts of the body to be affected by frostbite. An extremely low atmospheric temperature will cause pain in the extremities of the body until they become frozen. At this stage the skin is white and shining and then pain ceases. Because of this, the victim of frostbite may be unaware of its occurrence, and prolonged exposure may lead to necrosis of tissue. As thawing of the part takes place the surface blood vessels dilate once more and if this is sudden, the pain may be intense. The engorgement is followed by stasis of blood in the capillaries, exudation of serum and the formation of blisters, very similar to the injury caused by burns.

Treatment.—The first step in the treatment of frost-bite is the *very gradual* restoration of warmth and normal circulation in the part. This is best achieved by keeping the patient in a moderately warm room. Heat must not be applied to the nose, nor must the patient be allowed near the fire. The later treatment of the frost-bitten area is similar to that of burns.

An ointment containing sulphathiazole or penicillin may be applied on sterile dressings. Pain is relieved by analgesia.

Syphilis of the Nose

A primary syphilitic chancre on the nose is almost unknown, but secondary syphilis may produce lesions around the alæ at the same time as on other parts of the body. Infants suffering from congenital syphilis frequently develop mucous patches which extend into the nasal cavity and cause "snuffles". Gummatous destruction of bone tissue may give rise to a depression of the bridge of the nose, known as "saddle nose". This usually appears at about one year of age.

Tertiary syphilis may manifest itself as firm, painless nodules or as gummatous ulcers with deep sharp-cut edges which, when healed, leave soft, smooth, whitish scars described as "tissue paper". These ulcers are very destructive and common sites for them are about the nasal apertures and the lips.

Treatment.—The method of treatment of syphilis is the injection of penicillin procaine.

New Growths of the Nose

Small benign growths such as papillomata (warts) and angiomata (nævi) may occur on the nose and be removed, if desirable, by cautery or diathermy. The most common malignant growth of the nose is carcinoma.

Epithelioma, or Squamous-celled Carcinoma.—The first sign is the formation of small, waxy nodules or warts which gradually extend or deepen. Ulceration of the centre occurs, with crusting and bleeding. The edge of the ulcer is raised and rolled out. If the growth is allowed to develop, it may penetrate the nose. External irradiation, radium therapy or removal by scalpel or diathermy knife under local anæsthetic are the common methods of treatment. Healing after excision takes several weeks, and if the growth has penetrated to the mucous membrane, plastic surgery may be needed later.

Rodent Ulcer—Basal-celled Carcinoma.—This growth arises from cells in the sebaceous glands of the hair follicles or from the basal cells in the epidermis and most commonly develops on the face. A common site is at the entrance to the nostrils. They may be mistaken for simple inflammatory lesions, and careful examination is necessary. The base of the rodent ulcer is depressed and crusted, and the edge is pearly and slightly raised—the "rolled edge". Rodent ulcers develop slowly and are curable if diagnosed early. They are only locally malignant and do not invade the lymphatic system. The treatment is by irradiation or excision.

Foreign Bodies in the Nose

A foreign body has been defined as a substance not normally connected with its surroundings. Peas, beans and other small objects are commonly pushed into the nose by children without causing grave emergency. However, since the removal without causing further damage is difficult, such patients should be taken to a doctor or a hospital.

Foreign bodies remaining impacted in the nose give rise to discharge on the affected side, either of blood or pus. If the foreign body is seen to be smooth and rounded, the simplest method of removal is to pass a blunt-pointed director along the floor of the nose, under and behind the object and then gently withdraw it. Should the object be jagged or firmly impacted, the surgeon must remove it. The nose should be cocainized. Adrenaline may be added to the solution in order to cause shrinkage of the mucous membrane. Sometimes a general anæsthetic is given. Removal of the object is effected with forceps using a nasal speculum under good illumination.

Broken Nose, and Soft Tissue Wounds of the Face

In a direct blow on the face, the nose usually takes the main brunt of the force. The weak nasal bones readily yield, and the walls of the sinuses may give way if the violence is great. There is considerable bruising and swelling, and usually hæmorrhage from the nose. The first-aid treatment must avoid direct interference—there must be no blowing of the nose, douching or packing. Alternate hot and cold bathing may relieve pain and swelling. Later, after radiographs have been taken, the surgeon will reduce the fracture.

Any wounds of the soft tissues of the face should receive early treatment. All dirt must be removed and debris cleared. Systemic chemotherapy is advisable.

Epistaxis, or Nose Bleeding

Bleeding from the nose is one of the most common forms of hæmorrhage. It occurs especially in children and the elderly, very rarely in infants. The causes are legion, more often local than general disorders.

Causes.—Of the local disorders, the more common are: (*a*) injury, (*b*) superficial ulceration of inflammatory origin.

Among the general disorders, the commonest cause is a

DISEASES OF THE NOSE

raised blood pressure. Blood diseases such as leukæmia, anæmia, hæmophilia will also cause frequent epistaxis.

The bleeding in almost every case begins from a point on the septum called Kiesselbach's or Little's area, about a quarter of an inch inside the vestibule. At this spot is a very rich supply of blood vessels, both arteries and veins, whose thin walls readily become eroded.

Apart from the underlying causes and some head injuries, epistaxis is rarely serious. In most instances, it ceases spontaneously in a few minutes.

Treatment.—The first-aid treatment consists of pressure. The patient can immediately nip his own nose. Usually the bleeding is from one nostril only, though this is not always apparent at first. At the start the patient should blow his nose to clear loose clots. He should sit on a chair by a table and be given a pad of absorbent wool to hold against the nose. The elbow of the side that is bleeding should rest on the table. The nose can then be pressed against the thumb in an easy and comfortable position. The opposite nostril is free for respiratory purposes and, the head being kept forward, blood is not so liable to trickle down the pharynx.

Only too often, patients have been advised to hold the head back—this causes blood to be swallowed and results in nausea and vomiting, an unnecessary and distressing complication, which leads to further bleeding.

The patient may be given a cork or something similar to bite on. With a cork in the mouth he cannot easily swallow or breathe through his nose or move his palate. This puts the nose at rest and discourages bleeding.

When epistaxis does not spontaneously cease, the nose is packed with ribbon gauze impregnated with liquid paraffin to which has been added iodoform paste (see page 28). The packing may be left in place for several days if the patient is given antibiotic "cover" but is usually removed after 24 hours. An application of a 1 in 10,000 solution of venom from Russell's viper usually causes immediate clotting but is only useful if the bleeding point can be seen. Adrenaline solution may temporarily constrict vessels, but as its effect wears off, bleeding is apt to recur.

Morphine is ordered in severe cases for rest and sleep. The nurse should record the pulse rate and blood pressure every half hour, and give an estimate of the blood loss. Transfusion of blood may be needed.

In cases of bleeding at intervals, if the bleeding point can be easily seen and dealt with, a cautery may be used to seal the vessel. A swab of cotton wool, soaked in 10 per cent. cocaine solution (or 25 per cent. cocaine paste) is first applied to the bleeding point. After cauterization, the patient must be warned not to blow his nose for 3 days.

Very rarely, when epistaxis cannot be arrested by other means, ligation of the external carotid or ethmoidal artery is necessary.

Diseases of the Nasal Septum

Deviation of the Septum.—The septum is seldom a simple straight partition dividing the cavity. The deviation may be congenital or it may be due to injury. Frequently a blow or fall at an early age, unnoticed at the time or quickly forgotten, may cause bending of the cartilage which then ossifies crookedly. The perpendicular plate of the ethmoid bone is often markedly to one side so that it almost touches the middle turbinate and then it will interfere with the ventilation and drainage of the sinuses. Cartilaginous deviation is in the interior portion of the nose and is usually obvious on sight. It often involves the upper part of the quadrilateral cartilage. With severe injury the cartilage may be destroyed or project into the opposite nostril. Injuries in later life, especially if repeated as in boxing, may cause great irregularity so that both sides of the nose become obstructed.

Bony or cartilaginous outgrowths, called "spurs", may occur on the septum but these seldom give rise to symptoms of nasal obstruction. When the septum is deflected very much to one side, a large cavity is left in the opposite nostril, and the inferior turbinate then enlarges (see Fig. 19), which makes correction more complicated.

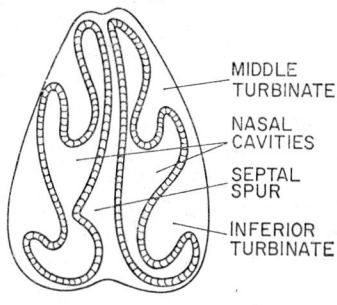

Fig. 19.—Deviation of the Nasal Septum (Diagrammatic).

When deviation of the septum is sufficient to cause nasal obstruction on either side, the mucous membrane becomes congested and œdematous. The openings from the sinuses become blocked, and, owing to stagnation of the secretion and consequent infection, the patients are particularly liable to colds and to sinusitis. Correction of the deformity is by surgery (see Submucous Resection of the Septum, page 88), but not as a rule under eighteen years of age, lest the nasal bridge should collapse for lack of the support normally provided by the septum.

Hæmatoma of the Septum.—This is a collection of blood between the layers of the septum usually due to injury. There may be external bruising and tenderness over the bridge of the nose, but the chief symptom is partial or complete nasal obstruction on both sides of the nose. The condition is diagnosed by inspection and palpation, or a diagnostic puncture may be made.

Treatment.—A hæmatoma often becomes infected and necrosis of cartilage will follow. Therefore, incision near the floor of the nose, on both sides of the septum if necessary, is advisable. The incision is made with a narrow-bladed knife under local anæsthesia, the blood clot is evacuated and a small drain of ribbon gauze is inserted.

Abscess of the Septum.—The usual cause of abscess of the septum is secondary infection of a hæmatoma, but abscesses occasionally follow an acute infection such as measles or typhoid fever, or are due to upward spread from a decayed incisor tooth root. The signs of suppuration are pyrexia, swelling and throbbing pain. The nose is slightly swollen and the skin is red and shining especially over the bridge and tip.

Treatment.—As soon as fluctuation is apparent, there should be incision of the abscess as described for hæmatoma. Sulphonamide powder may be dusted into the abscess cavity, and an antibiotic given systemically. It may be necessary to reinsert ribbon gauze daily for a few days to keep up free drainage. A small roll of sterile gauze may be fastened under the nose to absorb drainage and the patient's upper lip should be protected by ointment.

Complications.—The abscess usually takes about a week to heal leaving no after-effects, but occasionally perforation of the septum occurs, and necrosis is comparatively common. Necrosis leads to collapse of the nasal tip.

DISEASES OF THE NOSE

Perforation of the Septum.—This may follow various ulcerating diseases affecting the nose, or suppuration, injury, and particularly, inveterate nose-picking. The perforation may be quite symptomless, or a whistling sound may be present on either inspiration or expiration.

Treatment.—The treatment is that of the disease. Plastic repair may be performed.

Inflammatory Conditions of the Nose

Acute Catarrhal Rhinitis or Coryza.—These are synonymous terms applied to the inflammation of the mucous membrane of the nose known as the "common cold" which has already been discussed to some extent in Chapter 1. There is irritation of the mucous membrane producing sneezing, with dilatation of the mucus-secreting glands (goblet cells) and of blood vessels. At first the discharge consists of clear mucus, and after 12 to 24 hours, the nose becomes obstructed by the swollen mucous membrane. The eyes often water as the inflammation spreads up the lacrimal duct, and there is headache and malaise. These symptoms are due to many types of virus. Secondary bacterial infection commonly leads to further symptoms:

1. Purulent rhinitis, the nasal discharge becoming purulent and thick.
2. Sinusitis.
3. Laryngitis and cough, due to post-nasal discharge.

The acute stage of a cold lasts from 2 days to 1 week, after which the symptoms subside and the nasal mucous membrane returns to normal in 1 to 3 weeks. The temperature rarely rises above 37°C (99°F).

Acute rhinitis must be closely observed whenever it occurs during an epidemic. In *scarlet fever*, the temperature rises sharply to about 39°C (102°F) and there is marked sore throat and backache. A rash appears on the second day of the illness. In *measles*, Koplik's spots appear inside the cheeks on the second day. On the third day the temperature rises to about 39.5°C (103°F) and on the fourth day the rash appears. With *influenza,* there is more general malaise with aching of the limbs, and fewer nasal symptoms.

The principles to be followed are:
1. Isolation of the patient.
2. Relief of symptoms.
3. Prevention of secondary infection.

Treatment of Acute Rhinitis.—At the onset of a cold, it is in the patient's own interest and that of others that he should go to bed. Aspirin and copious fluids, preferably hot, will relieve the headache and sore throat.

After a day or two, symptoms subside and treatment may be reduced. The nose must be kept clear of discharge and crusts, and all coughs and sneezes guarded by a handkerchief. The correct use and treatment of handkerchiefs has already been mentioned. It is advisable to smear the upper lip and around the vestibule of the nose with a mild ointment to prevent cracks.

Herpes Simplex, or "cold sores" frequently appear around the mouth following a cold. The predisposing cause is a virus which resides in the skin of certain individuals whose tendency to herpes is aggravated by any condition causing irritation. Vesicles occur on the lips and cause constant "tickling" discomfort. After about 24 hours the vesicles rupture and crusts are formed. If left alone, healing rapidly takes place. But if the patient succumbs to the great temptation to pick off irritating crusts this leads to bleeding areas and delay in recovery.

Treatment.—Since herpes simplex is so common, the remedies advocated are legion. Most sufferers have their favourite applications. A quickly drying ointment with a basis of zinc oxide or collodion, applied to the lip at the onset of discomfort may avert or limit the outbreak, and a spirituous application to the ulcer will relieve pain and hasten the healing.

DISEASES OF THE NOSE

Chronic Rhinitis.—Recurrent attacks of acute rhinitis, due to some underlying cause which prevents free drainage of the nose, lead to permanent changes in the nasal mucosa, and then the condition becomes chronic. Such causes are, commonly, disease of the paranasal sinuses, adenoids, or deviation of the nasal septum, and less commonly, occupation in a dusty atmosphere. Sometimes, however, no cause is found.

There are several types of chronic rhinitis.

Chronic Hypertrophic Rhinitis.—In this type, the mucous membrane, especially over the posterior part of the inferior turbinate process is thick and œdematous. There is an abnormal secretion of thin sticky mucus. The patient cannot breathe through the nose, and mouth breathing leads frequently to pharyngitis and laryngitis. There is constant headache and lassitude. When treated with vasoconstrictors, the mucous membrane fails to shrink completely, as there is dilatation and thickening of the blood vessels, enlargement of the mucous glands and interstitial fibrosis. The treatment consists of removing the cause; sinusitis may be treated, deviation of the septum corrected. The patient is advised to avoid smoking and alcohol. Cauterization may be employed to contract the thickened mucosa.

Chronic Atrophic Rhinitis.—This is a disappearing disease. It becomes evident at puberty, and the sufferers are often women who have been undernourished in the past. Its cause is probably connected with some neglected infection. There is drying, shrinking and fibrosis of the mucous membrane, followed by atrophy of the turbinate bones so that the nasal fossæ appear particularly spacious, and the nasopharynx can easily be seen. The mucosa is pale. The patient complains of constant crust-formation in the nose. The crusts are greenish and may become very offensive, when the condition is known as ozœna. The foul odour (which is often unnoticed by the patient herself, since the sense of smell is lost), is thought to be due to the invasion of bacilli which, however, do not cause the atrophy.

Treatment. The nostrils must be kept as clean as possible. Saline irrigations are used, and once daily this may be followed by spraying the nose with œstrogen in oil. The œstrogen may be gradually reduced to weekly or fortnightly treatment, or a watery solution of glucose and glycerine may be used.

Allergic Rhinitis—Hay Fever.—Allergy of the respiratory mucous membrane is usually due to irritation from pollen (especially of grasses, hence its common title), household or occupational dust, cosmetics containing orris root, and moulds. The condition may be complicated by food allergy.

The symptoms are irritation in the anterior nares, violent sneezing, watery nasal discharge, and often streaming eyes. The nose is obstructed, the mucous membrane being typically pale and œdematous, although it occasionally appears normal or slightly red. When a specimen of the nasal discharge is stained and examined in the laboratory, eosinophils (acid-staining leucocytes) are found to be present in large numbers. Other manifestations of allergy, such as asthma or urticaria, may point to a diagnosis.

Skin tests are made by scratch or intradermal injection to discover the particular sensitivity of individual patients, such substances being used as the extracts of foodstuffs, pollens, and the dandruff of animals. When tests have shown the origin of the allergy, diluted extract of the offending material is injected subcutaneously in order to desensitize the patient. Slowly increasing doses at weekly intervals are given early in the year. If too big a dose is given, intense hay-fever symptoms and severe urticaria occur. These are relieved by antihistamine tablets. Pure "hay fever" is caused only by pollen. Should the cause of the allergy be undetected, injections of mixed proteins may be tried.

DISEASES OF THE NOSE

Treatment.—Antihistamic drugs such as Phenergan, Thephorin and Piriton provide great relief when given by mouth, three times daily. Otherwise little can be done for the patient at the time of the attack which lasts intermittently for several days, except to relieve the exhaustion caused by the violent sneezing. The sufferer should avoid over-heating—either by a fire or too warm bedclothes, as this intensifies the symptoms.

The electric cautery or diathermy may be applied to the inferior turbinate processes if there is hypertrophy in the obstinate, chronic, non-seasonal case, but unless there is marked deformity, operation should be avoided.

Miscellaneous Conditions of the Nose

Nasal Polypi.—These are benign overgrowths of fibrovascular tissue which develop from the œdematous mucous membrane caused by nasal allergy or long-standing infection. The polypi are large greyish masses, usually multiple, and have the appearance of a bunch of grapes. They are usually pedunculated and project into the nose, sometimes appearing at the anterior nares. Polypi most often arise in the ethmoid sinuses, sometimes from the middle turbinates, or from the antra, and may cause marked obstruction, a nasal voice and headaches.

They may block the posterior nares, when they are called choanal polypi. Occasionally the surface of polypi may become ulcerated or hæmorrhagic, respectively causing purulent discharge or epistaxis.

Treatment.—Occasionally a polypus is blown out of the nose, or disappears, but surgical removal with a snare is usually required. Unless the underlying cause can be removed, polypi will recur.

Tuberculosis of the Nasal Cavity.—*Lupus vulgaris* (see page 66) may spread from the skin around the vestibule into the nasal cavity. It causes severe ulceration and destruction of the soft parts of the nose. There is a subacute variety manifesting flat pale vegetations which break down into ulcers. There is usually no ozœna, and the condition may be confined to the nasal cavity for a long time.

Treatment.—Blood tests are made to exclude syphilis, and microscopic examination of a small portion of mucous membrane may be made to confirm the diagnosis. A strict régime for the general treatment of tuberculosis is necessary until the disease is under control. The warty growths may be coagulated by diathermy, or cautery, or application of chromic acid, after crusts have been removed by a mild alkaline solution. Patients must be encouraged to keep up outpatient attendance long after apparent cure.

Nasal Diphtheria—Membranous Rhinitis.—There are times when the Corynebacterium diphtheriae will attack the nose as a primary infection without affecting the larynx. The patient is not as a rule acutely ill. There is nasal obstruction and a sudden, unilateral blood-stained discharge, and on examination, a greyish-white membrane can sometimes be seen on the inferior turbinate bone and adjacent parts. When the membrane is removed, a bleeding area is left.

Treatment.—As soon as the disease is recognized, without waiting for laboratory tests, the patient is isolated, given antitoxin, and arrangements are made for him to be removed to an infectious-diseases hospital. (See also pages 115–116 for faucial diphtheria and page 146 for laryngeal diphtheria.)

Choanal Atresia.—In this rare condition, which may be congenital or acquired, the posterior nares are blocked by membrane or bone. If acquired, it is due to injury or to severe infection, such as diphtheria or tuberculosis, followed by scarring. The chief symptom of atresia is the absence of breathing in the affected side.

When the condition is congenital and bilateral, it is noticed from birth that the child is unable to breathe and suck at the same time. Examination reveals the blockage. Surgical removal of the obstructing membrane or bone is required. It can be a matter of great urgency in the newborn child if the condition is bilateral, owing to difficulty with breathing and feeding.

9

Diseases of the paranasal sinuses

Acute Maxillary Sinusitis

When considering this condition, it is as well to remember that in a young child, the second dentition in the maxillary bones develops at a short distance below the orbits. The descent of the teeth is due to the laying down of new bone. Some air spaces are present in the bone at birth, and these increase in size, eventually forming the large maxillary air sinuses or antra. At nine years of age the floor of the maxillary sinus is at the same level as the floor of the nose. The sinus is fully formed when the third molars (wisdom teeth) are cut—that is at about the twenty-fifth year. It then extends from the second premolar to the third molar tooth, upwards to the floor of the orbit, and sideways to the wall of the nose at the level of the inferior turbinate (see Fig. 1). Above this, in the wall of the middle meatus, is the ostium into the nose from the sinus. A small accessory opening is often found in front of and below the ostium. The inferior orbital nerve crosses the roof of the maxillary sinus and the superior alveolar nerve lies in its floor.

Symptoms.—Acute infection of the maxillary sinus is usually a sequel to acute rhinitis due to spread by continuity through the maxillary ostium or the accessory opening, or may result from infection of a tooth root in the floor of the sinus. The chief predisposing factor is a blocked middle meatus. Pain and tenderness occur in the cheek, in the teeth on the affected side, and over the eye. The last symptom may imply involvement of the frontal sinus.

Treatment.—The initial treatment is that of an ordinary cold. Pain may be relieved by analgesics, and by heat in the form of either a steam inhalation or an external application. The attack often disappears spontaneously, but should the symptoms be severe, penicillin is often given. Should pain and discharge continue then a trocar and cannula can be passed into the nose and the wall between the sinus and nose punctured (antrum, or proof puncture, see page 91), and the sinus irrigated. Occasionally a permanent opening in the wall of the inferior meatus is needed (intranasal antrostomy).

With a subacute infection, suction displacement therapy (see page 30) with ephedrine or penicillin solution may cure the condition.

Chronic Maxillary Sinusitis

Signs.—Recurrent attacks of acute sinusitis, or an acute attack which fails to resolve will become a chronic condition. There is persistent nasal and postnasal discharge, but no fever. On examination, pus can be seen in the middle meatus and on the back wall of the pharynx. The diagnosis is confirmed by transillumination and X-ray appearances.

Treatment.—Every factor which might hinder free drainage of the sinus should receive attention. Polypi should be removed, a deviated septum should be corrected. These measures may be sufficient, but if necessary repeated antrum irrigation should be performed. Operation should be undertaken only when the lining membrane of the antrum is irreversibly altered, i.e. shows itself incapable of return to the normal state. Caldwell-Luc's operation (see page 93) is a radical removal of the thickened mucous membrane, and this operation is replacing the intranasal antrostomy in many centres.

Frontal Sinusitis

Since the frontal sinuses are late in developing, inflammation of them is not found under six years of age.

Some inflammation of the frontal sinus may occur with maxillary sinusitis and may persist as chronic frontal sinusitis.

Symptoms.—The patient complains of heaviness and tenderness over the eyes and inability to concentrate. Frontal headache is usual. As a rule, it is absent on rising, comes on during the morning, reaching its maximum at noon, and has gone by tea time. If the pain does not lessen at night, the conclusion is that natural drainage of the sinus is absent. There is often copious discharge. The discharge is most marked on rising, and, on examination, pus can be seen to cover the thickened mucous membrane in the middle meatus of the nose. The frontal sinus is opaque in a radiograph.

Nasal polypi are sometimes present. Obstruction of the naso-frontal duct may give rise to a mucocele—a cyst in the sinus containing mucus. This must be completely removed as it may become infected, or increase in size and erode the orbit.

Treatment.—All patients with acute frontal sinusitis should be in bed. The treatment of the accompanying maxillary sinusitis (see page 83) may provide better drainage. If these measures do not relieve the patient's distress, then a small burr-hole is made into the floor of the frontal sinus and a drainage tube is inserted.

Ethmoidal Sinusitis

A patient who suffers from maxillary or frontal sinusitis has always an associated inflammation of the ethmoid sinuses. In a child, the ethmoid sinusitis may be the presenting disease in an acute case.

Symptoms.—These are largely obscured by those of the maxillary or frontal sinusitis.

Treatment.—This is included in that of the larger affected sinus and is usually conservative. In infants, however, where the infection presents as swelling, incision and drainage may be needed.

Sphenoidal Sinusitis

Inflammation of the sphenoid sinus is very uncommon but as a rule responds quickly to simple treatment.

Symptoms.—The headache in this condition differentiates it from the other forms of sinus infections with which it is associated. There is occipital pain which may spread over the mastoid process, and there may be pain at the back of the eye. Other symptoms of acute sphenoid sinusitis are stiffness of the neck muscles; vague unsteadiness, which may be continuous or intermittent, and is increased on turning the head; sleeplessness due chiefly to periodic discharge from the sinus into the throat; dryness at the back of the nose and a persistent, tickling, throaty cough. The discharge is thick and can be seen coming from behind the palate.

If chronic sphenoid sinusitis supervenes, the headache becomes continuous, and is increased on exercise, smoking or drinking alcohol. Toxæmia may cause mental depression and inability to concentrate. Ocular symptoms such as exophthalmos and visual disturbances occur late. A dry throat is typical.

Complications.—The complications of severe untreated acute sphenoid sinusitis are likely to be serious. That most to be feared is cavernous sinus thrombosis (see page 66). Partial or complete blindness may develop.

Treatment.—The acute case is treated by antibiotics. Very rarely is anything further needed. The chronic case may be treated by removing the antero-inferior sinus wall. To achieve this, part of the septum may need resection.

Paranasal Tumours

New growths of the paranasal sinuses are uncommon, but are more often malignant than benign. They are usually carcinomata arising from the ethmoid or the maxillary antrum. The growth may extend into the nose (causing unilateral obstruction, discharge and epistaxis), into the orbit (displacing the eye), downwards into the hard palate, or outwards causing swelling of the cheek. Pain is characteristic.

The treatment consists of irradiation followed by wide removal of involved bone.

10

Surgical operations on the nose and paranasal sinuses

Preparation of the Patient

The general preparation of a patient for a nasal operation is as for any other surgical operation. The patient's heart, lungs and urine are examined. X-ray photographs of the sinuses will be taken, and bacteriological examinations made of nose and throat swabs. The operation is postponed if the patient is suffering from an acute infection—for example, coryza, tonsillitis or acute sinusitis. Starvation increases the tendency to vomiting and most patients can be given a normal, but easily digested diet, up to 6 hours before operation (unless other directions are given). Sugar often in the form of glucose is valuable, especially for diabetics, as a good store of glycogen in the liver helps to prevent post-operative acidosis which is a cause of vomiting. Children will usually take barley sugar readily and this is a quickly assimilable sugar. A patient is well advised to refrain from smoking for 24 hours before operation.

The local preparation consists of cleaning the vestibule of the nose, the mouth and the upper lip. Some surgeons prefer the lip shaved. If not, any moustache must be washed carefully and the lip rendered as clean as possible. Immediately before the operation, the patient is given a mouthwash. Patients will usually be ordered a pre-operative sedative.

Nasal operations are performed under local or general anæsthesia. For both types, the nose is sprayed and gauze-packed with 10 per cent. cocaine solution, or it is painted with 25 per cent. cocaine paste, or postural instillation of cocaine may be adopted. In the last case the cocaine solution is instilled into the nose with the patient in various positions—right lateral, knee-elbow and left lateral positions for 5 minutes each. The nurse should explain to the patient the reasons for this exercise.

Submucous Resection of the Septum

The patient is made comfortable, either sitting up or lying on the operating table, with head and shoulders slightly raised on a pillow. If local anæsthetic is used the eyes are bandaged or covered with a sterile towel which is placed under the head in the theatre. The patient is reassured and encouraged to relax with the hands lying flat and limp at his sides. The sterile towels are then secured to cover the patient's body completely from toes to chin and over the head and eyes. The nasal packs are withdrawn and the skin of the nose and upper lip are mopped with a skin-sterilizing agent.

To supplement the pre-operative cocainization, the surgeon may inject 1 in 1000 Nupercaine solution or Xylocaine into the mucous membrane on each side of the septum. He makes an incision with a small sharp-pointed knife on one side of the septum. The mucous membrane is then lifted with a flat-sided elevator from the cartilage and bone on that side. Next, the septal cartilage is incised and the mucous membrane elevated on the other side, great care being taken to avoid perforating this layer of mucous membrane. The surgeon then removes a portion of the cartilage and bone. Any bony spurs are removed with a sharp elevator or a fish-tail gouge and mallet. When the airway is perfectly clear, the septal flaps of mucous membrane are replaced to meet. It is usual to pack each nostril in order to keep the two layers of membrane together and prevent blood clot forming between them. The packing may be done with ribbon gauze soaked in liquid paraffin, or with rubber finger-stalls stuffed with gauze and lubricated with petroleum jelly, or some form of nasal splint. Stitching is usually not required. It is customary to place a wool filament gauze bolster under the external nares and secure it with adhesive.

FIG. 20.—NASAL BOLSTER.

After-treatment.—The patient must not on any account blow his nose for fear of causing bleeding and hæmatoma. Sterile gauze swabs are provided for mopping any blood that oozes from the nostrils. The nurse should find out from the surgeon when the nasal packs, if any, are to be removed. (In special cases they may be left 24 or even 48 hours.). The patient should lie quietly for half an hour after removal of the pack to prevent hæmorrhage and should remain more or less in bed 2 or 3 days.

Four-hourly steam inhalations, usually with tincture of benzoin, are given as routine treatment, preceded by drops of mild silver protein (Protargol) and ephedrine drops. When, in approximately 1 week, the patient is discharged from hospital, he is recommended for 2 weeks' holiday and should be warned against violent exercise for at least a week. Should epistaxis occur, he should report to the hospital, as great care must be taken to prevent hæmatoma of the septum.

The method of compressing the septum to arrest epistaxis should be taught him before he is discharged from the ward (see page 71). Patients should be warned that relief from nasal obstruction will not be immediate and is delayed for some weeks, till healing has been completed.

Removal of Nasal Polypi

This operation is frequently performed in the outpatients' department, but is often combined with other operations on the nasal sinuses. If the patient has many polypi, or if sinus infection is present, the patient is admitted to the ward, and after operation is kept in bed for 2 or 3 days and treated with menthol or friars' balsam inhalations.

To remove the polypi, the nose is cocainized. A wire snare is passed round the base of each lobule of polypus which is avulsed. Before sterilizing the snare, the nurse should ensure that the wire is unbroken and the loop is straight. Small polypi may be removed with Luc's forceps. If there is much bleeding, the nose is packed, but usually a little cotton wool to mop up any drops of blood is sufficient.

Cauterization of the Nose

A galvanocautery handle and points and a nasal speculum are required. The cautery is usually heated by a transformer from the mains. When the nose has been anæsthetized, the current is turned on until the point warms to a bright red. It is then applied to the tissues round the bleeding point. The cautery is removed from the nose before the current is turned off and the cautery point is cleaned by passing the current through it until all secretions are burned away. It is then detached from the handle and put away. After cauterization, the patient is given some ointment to apply to the nostril daily until the area is healed.

Proof Puncture of the Maxillary Sinus (Intranasal Antrotomy or Antral Puncture)

The patient is prepared by having the inferior meatus of the affected side cocainized. A Lichtwitz trocar and cannula is inserted into the inferior meatus and the wall of the sinus is pierced at a point about 2.5 cm from

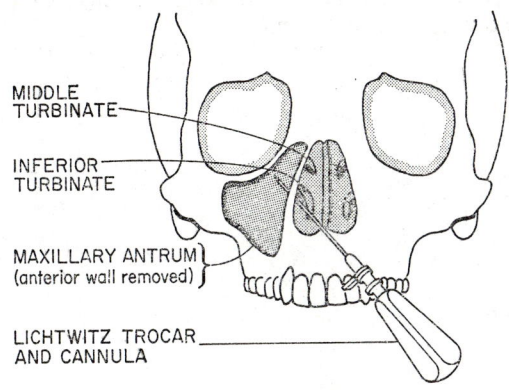

FIG. 21.—ANTRAL PUNCTURE.

the anterior end of the turbinate process. The trocar is then withdrawn leaving the cannula in position. A 10 ml syringe which contains 3 or 4 ml of normal saline is fitted to the Lichtwitz cannula. The plunger of the syringe is withdrawn to aspirate the fluid contents of the cavity. If nothing is obtained, the saline is injected and withdrawn from the sinus. Pus may be obtained, of which a specimen is sent to the pathological laboratory for examination. If return of fluid does not follow the injection of saline, it is probable that the sinus is full of polypoid tissue, or that the needle has penetrated too far. If the proof puncture is positive, and purulent fluid is returned, a Higginson's syringe can be attached to the cannula and the sinus washed out. The Higginson's syringe must be quite full of fluid before it is attached. The fluid passes through the natural ostium of the sinus, into the nose, and then out into a receiver held under the patient's chin.

After irrigation, a small quantity of $\frac{1}{2}$ per cent. ephedrine in normal saline, or of penicillin fluid or other appropriate antibiotic is sometimes injected into the cavity, through the cannula.

Fig. 22.—Polythene Tube in Right Maxillary Sinus.

As a rule, the patient is kept at rest in the outpatients' waiting room for half an hour after the operation, and may then go home. A little oozing of blood-stained serum is to be expected for two or three days.

Sometimes the surgeon decides on a daily antral

washout for a week or so. To avoid repeated puncture, a fine polythene tube may be passed through the cannula into the antrum and left in position on withdrawing the cannula. The tube is fastened to the nose and forehead with strapping, and through it irrigation or the instillation of penicillin fluid can easily be carried out. This method is used especially for children thus avoiding repeated general anæsthetics.

Intranasal Antrostomy (Antral Window)

This operation establishes a temporary or permanent opening into the maxillary sinus to permit repeated lavage when medical treatment and proof puncture have failed to cure subacute sinusitis. The anterior end of the inferior turbinate bone is dislocated upwards, or, if necessary, is removed with punch forceps, and an opening through the wall of the sinus is made with a trephine or other perforating instrument. The opening is made as low and as far forward as possible. It is enlarged with biting forceps and an antrum chisel. Pus usually wells out of the sinus at this stage. The cavity is washed out and the ephedrine or penicillin injected as for simple antral puncture.

Radical Antrostomy (Caldwell-Luc's Operation)

When the mucous membrane is grossly infected, or when polypi are present in the maxillary sinus, the whole lining must be removed. The approach to the antrum is under the upper lip, in the canine fossa. No pre-operative packing is required, but the nose is usually cocainized before the operation.

Sometimes the operation is performed under general anæsthesia given by the intratracheal route. The postnasal space and the pharynx can then be packed to prevent blood and secretions from entering the trachea.

If general anæsthesia is required, the patient is usually given a pre-operative hypodermic injection of atropine sulphate 0.6 mg. Before a local anæsthetic, papaverine (Omnopon) 30–40 mg is given.

When the patient is on the operation table, either the local or the general anæsthetic is supplemented by Nupercaine ½ or 1 per cent. with adrenaline 1 in 1000 in the proportion of 0.3 ml of adrenaline in 30 ml. This, the anæsthetist injects into the area of the incision, above the canine and the first and second molar teeth. If the patient is unconscious, the mouth may be lightly packed with gauze. The upper lip being well retracted, the surgeon makes his incision, and then, with dental drill or hammer and gouge makes the opening into the antrum. If much bleeding occurs, 1 ml of adrenaline solution is applied on a swab into the cavity. The opening is enlarged with nibbling forceps until the inside of the sinus is visible. Suction apparatus is essential so that the field of operation can be kept clear of blood and purulent fluid. The antral cavity is cleared of diseased mucous membrane and a new opening into the nose is made beneath the inferior turbinate.

A section of the mucous membrane is usually sent to the pathological laboratory for examination. Usually the sinus is left unpacked. A certain amount of oozing of blood and serum is expected for 2 or 3 days, and when the opening is no longer required it soon heals. Some surgeons close, or partly close the mouth wound with three or four interrupted catgut sutures—these do not need removal—or with wire sutures, which are removed on the fourth day.

Complications.—In the case of severe post-operative bleeding, the antrum is irrigated with saline solution at 44°C (110°F), and the nose may need packing. When it is certain that the bleeding has ceased, the packing is removed by the house surgeon or ward sister.

Patients who are bleeding or restless are given morphine 16 mg. Also, an aspirin mixture may be given to relieve headache. After operation some patients complain of neuralgia or anæsthesia of the face for a few days, but this is temporary only and they should be reassured on this point. Frequently swelling of the face occurs and this may be treated by the application of external heat. It usually disappears in 4 or 5 days.

Sometimes the eyes become black and swollen. If so, a petroleum jelly pad and a pressure bandage may be applied overnight. The swelling will have subsided by the morning.

A more lasting complication is fistula into the mouth. This may be due to the previous removal of a tooth which has caused suppuration and left a patent tooth socket. The treatment is plastic repair.

After-treatment.—After all operations on the nose and sinuses, strict attention to the mouth toilet is essential. Routine syringing of the antrum is not now commonly practised, but is occasionally ordered if marked sepsis exists. Menthol inhalations and nasal drops may be given 4-hourly. Dentures may be reworn as soon as the patient finds them comfortable. The antrostomy opening into the nose contracts, but does not close completely.

An operation similar to the Caldwell-Luc is performed to remove a tumour of the antrum. A routine "cover" with a sulphonamide or antibiotic is usually ordered by the surgeon for 4 or 5 days.

Partial Ethmoidectomy

Intranasal Operation.—This is a simple procedure, frequently combined with other operations on the nose such as antrostomy or the removal of polypi. Under local anæsthesia, the diseased ethmoid cells are scraped out by means of a curette and punch forceps.

External Operation.—Before operation the eyebrow and skin area is carefully cleaned. A curved incision is made between the bridge of the nose and the eye. Before commencing the operation, the nose is cocainized on the side to be operated on, and both eyes are smeared with sterile petroleum jelly to prevent blood running into them.

After making the incision, the surgeon divides the structures down to the periosteum which is retracted. The ethmoid cells are curetted, and drainage is provided into the nose. The external wound is then closed with silkworm gut or silver wire sutures. A small drainage tube is inserted for 24 hours.

A petroleum jelly dressing and eye pad are bandaged firmly over the eye, using a fast-edged cotton bandage. The dressing is examined after 12 hours. If there is swelling, or if a tube has been used, a fresh dressing is applied for another 12 or 24 hours. The wound is then left uncovered and the patient is allowed out of bed. Stitches are removed after 4 days. Should the eye be infected, 10 per cent. sulphacetamide or appropriate antibiotic drops may be instilled four times daily.

Operations on the Frontal Sinus

External Operations.—The X-ray photographs of the frontal sinuses will indicate their exact size and position, and are therefore of great assistance in these operations.

The Trephine Operation.—This is performed for acute frontal sinusitis. The incision is made between the bridge of the nose and the eye and the tissues are divided down to the bone. In order to avoid penetrating the cancellous bone of the orbital ridge which might result in osteomyelitis, the entry is made through the compact bone forming the floor of the sinus. The opening is made large enough for a fairly rigid rubber tube, not less than 8 millimetres in diameter, to be inserted. A "portex" tube, made of plastic material, very smooth and resistant to pressure, is often used. As a rule, the pus drains through this under pressure. The tube is stitched to the skin. The sinus is irrigated through the tube and the fluid passes into the nose when the fronto-nasal duct reopens.

For chronic frontal sinusitis, there are various operations in practice.

Howarth's Operation.—The floor of the frontal sinus and part of the anterior ethmoid wall are removed forming a new channel into the nose.

Negus's Operation.—This is similar but the new channel into the nose is lined with a Thiersch graft to prevent adhesions and the narrowing of the opening by scar tissue.

Before all these operations, the preparation of the patient is similar to that described for external ethmoidectomy. The patient is most often given a general anæsthetic.

When the frontal sinus has been opened the fronto-nasal duct is widened and a plastic tube inserted. The latter is brought out through the nostril and left in place for many weeks according to the directions of the surgeon. It is important that the tube be left until fibrosis has ended. The external wound is closed with silkworm gut or silver wire sutures.

The dressing of the wound is similar to that for ethmoidectomy.

Obliteration of the Frontal Sinus.—Since this operation causes considerable deformity of the upper face, it is rarely performed except in an emergency or for osteomyelitis of the frontal bone. The operation involves the removal of the orbital ridge and the entire outer wall of the sinus.

The Osteoplastic Operation.—This has largely replaced the obliteration operation. An incision is made within the hairline after shaving the vault, and the anterior walls of the frontal sinuses are turned forwards attached to the scalp. The diseased lining and bone are removed, the ethmoids opened from above and the anterior wall of the sinuses replaced.

Operations for New Growth of Maxillary Antrum

Radiotherapy may precede or *follow* surgical treatment according to the decision of the surgeon and the radiotherapist in the light of the particular circumstances in each case.

(i) If the growth is small and of easy access, excision by the sublabial route (Caldwell Luc's) is carried out.

(ii) Following external irradiation, the nasal fossa and the maxillary sinus are exposed by removal of the bony walls, including the upper alveolus and hard palate. The growth is coagulated by diathermy and the debris removed. The cavity may be skin-grafted and packed. A bag of gauze may be used, containing strips soaked in iodoform. This is removed after about a week. A denture carrying an obturator to fill the defect is then inserted to prevent the soft tissues from contracting. If the palate is not involved, an attempt is made to preserve as much as possible in order to facilitate feeding and speech.

(iii) If the skin of the cheek or the deeper regions of the nose are affected, an external operation (lateral rhinotomy) is performed. This requires subsequent plastic repair.

Trans-sphenoidal Hypophysectomy

The removal of the hypophysis (pituitary gland) is an operation performed by ear, nose and throat surgeons. The great majority of hypophysectomies are for uncontrolled breast cancer, particularly when painful bony metastases are present, but the operation can also be used for other diseases. As far as breast cancer is concerned, it is not possible at present to decide in advance which growths are hormone-dependent. About one third of the patients have a remarkable relief from pain, usually lasting months; in another third painful bony metastases and ulcerating skin deposits disappear. In the latter group, the remission may last three or four years.

In trans-sphenoidal hypophysectomy, access is obtained via an external ethmoidectomy, or via the nose or by a combination of these routes. Excellent exposure is obtained without the risks of a major intracranial procedure or of optic nerve injury.

Pre-operative Management

The patient is admitted a few days before the operation, and a series of investigations are undertaken:—

Haemoglobin and blood count.

Blood grouping and cross-matching.

Blood sugar, blood urea and serum electrolytes.

X-rays of chest, skull and sinuses. These should be checked carefully for evidence of metastases, which might affect the type of incision.

Prophylactic antibiotics are commenced, e.g. penicillin 1 mega unit 6-hourly. A sulphonamide such as sulphadiazine 1 g 6-hourly may also be used. To combat the hormonal disturbance occasioned by the removal of the pituitary gland, cortisone therapy is begun. Hydrocortisone 100 mg can be given intramuscularly the night before operation and repeated during the morning before operation. If hypophysectomy is undertaken for intractable pain, the patient may be having a considerable amount of analgesia. This should be continued prior to surgery.

The patient should be given an explanation of the various investigations that are being carried out and she should understand the nature of the operation. Close relatives should also be told what is being undertaken and the expected result.

A muscle graft will be needed to pack the pituitary fossa, and for this purpose the right thigh is shaved and the skin cleansed with soap and water.

The anæsthetist usually sees the patient the day before operation, and prescribes a suitable pre-medication to be given 1 to 1½ hours before surgery. A hypnotic will be given to insure a good night's sleep prior to the operation.

At operation a blood transfusion is begun, and a further dose of hydrocortisone may be given. Muscle taken from the thigh is packed into the pituitary fossa with ribbon gauze soaked in liquid paraffin. The pack is brought out through the nose. Raytex ribbon gauze is used to distinguish it from the nasal packs. The wound is sutured. If the external ethmoidal approach is used, an eye pad and bandage may be applied on the affected side. If the nasal approach is made, a nasal splint is applied externally. This is made of gauze soaked in collodion. Both nostrils are packed with ribbon gauze. There is usually a moderate amount of bleeding.

Post-operative Management

Usually a general anæsthetic has been given and the patient is nursed flat on her side. The intravenous infusion is continued with Dextrose 4 per cent. in $\frac{1}{5}$ normal saline. As a rule, 2 bottles of blood are transfused during the operation. The nurse should observe the patient carefully, particularly noting the general condition, colour, and nature of the respirations. The pulse rate and blood pressure should be taken and recorded at ½-hourly intervals for the first few hours. If the systolic pressure falls below 100 mmHg, 100 mg hydrocortisone may be ordered and given intramuscularly. The patient usually continues to have hydrocortisone 6-hourly until she is able to take drugs orally. Then, Prednisolone 50 mg 6-hourly may be ordered instead. The antibiotics and sulphonamide are continued up to 12 days after operation. Analgesics are given as ordered and as required. An aspirin mixture given 4-hourly is found to be very useful and is usually sufficient to control any discomfort after the first 48 hours. A fluid balance chart should be maintained. There may be signs of diabetes insipidus but this can be controlled by intramuscular pitressin.

On the 1st day the eye pad is removed and the eyes are then bathed 4-hourly. The nasal packs are removed. The patient should be able to take sufficient fluid orally and the infusion can be discontinued. The patient should be nursed with her head raised on two pillows. She can lie on alternate sides or her back to relieve pressure areas. She may eat and drink whatever she can enjoy. The eyebrow incision sutures are removed about the 4th day, nasal sutures at the end of a week and the thigh sutures about the 10th day. The pituitary pack is removed after the 9th post-operative day. If there is no leak of cerebrospinal fluid, the patient begins to sit out of bed and gradually to walk about in the ward. Thyroid replacement is needed and a small dose of thyroxine taken orally, is commenced. The dose of Prednisolone is gradually reduced. Antibiotics should be discontinued.

Before discharge from hospital the patient should understand the importance of taking the drugs she has been prescribed and particularly the need to increase the dose of Prednisolone if she is under conditions of stress. She must therefore remain under close supervision of her doctor or the hospital.

Care of Patients who have had a General Anæsthetic for Operations on the Nose and Throat

In most cases of nose and throat operations performed under general anæsthesia, the amount of anæsthetic given is such that the patient is beginning to regain consciousness before leaving the theatre. This precaution is taken because, until the cough reflex returns, there is danger that blood may be inhaled and cause asphyxia or pneumonia. Until the patient is fully conscious, his head should be placed so that the tongue falls forward, leaving the airway clear so that vomit, mucus or blood drain freely from the mouth. To maintain a free airway by preventing the tongue from falling back into the pharynx the nurse should place her thumb, or first and second fingers, behind the angle of the patient's jaw and pull the jaw forward.

Fig. 23.—Post-Anæsthetic Tonsillectomy) Position.

Before leaving the table the patient is placed in the so-called "Tonsillectomy position". He is turned on his right side, the lower (i.e. right) knee is drawn up to form a supporting wedge and his right arm brought beneath his chin (see Fig. 23). This position is maintained during the return to the ward and until the patient recovers consciousness.

A tray beside the bed should contain gauze or gauze-covered swabs, sponge holders, tongue depressor, mouth gag, tongue forceps, a bowl of cold water, a receiver, vomit bowl and vomit towel. The bedclothes should be protected against staining by means of a plastic sheet and towel.

The nurse in charge of the patient, must keep a constant watch until consciousness has fully returned. She should notice his colour, breathing and pulse, keeping a ¼-hourly pulse chart. Noisy breathing denotes obstruction; cyanosis indicates a deficiency of oxygen; pallor, a rapid pulse and swallowing movements indicate bleeding. Should an artificial airway or mouth prop have been left in the mouth by the anæsthetist, this should not be removed until the patient is fully conscious as it prevents swallowing. Any sponge inserted during the operation should be left until the patient is conscious enough to spit it out.

The danger of shallow breathing should also be remembered as an important item to be observed by the nurse in charge of an anæsthetized patient. This condition, coupled with a slight degree of obstruction may lead to a state of dangerous anoxæmia (lack of oxygen in the blood). The treatment is to check the airway and give an inhalation of oxygen.

The nurse should realize that hearing is the last sense to disappear under anæsthetic and the first to return. Conversation should therefore be cautious and any remarks encouraging—for example, that the patient was very good or that the operation was successful.

Section III: The Pharynx

11

Anatomy of the pharynx

The nose and mouth open into the pharynx which is the common passage for food and air leading to the œsophagus and the larynx. The pharynx is divided into the nasopharynx, the oropharynx and the laryngeal pharynx.

The **Nasopharynx** lies above the soft palate and has five openings; the two posterior nares, the orifices of the two pharyngotympanic (Eustachian) tubes, and the opening downward into the oropharynx. The pharyngotympanic tubes are composed of cartilage lined by mucous membrane and at each orifice is a prominent bulge of the same tissues (see Fig. 14). On the roof of the nasopharynx in childhood, and sometimes persisting into adult life, is the pharyngeal tonsil, which, if enlarged, is known as adenoids.

The **Oropharynx** lies between the soft palate and the upper edge of the epiglottis. It opens above into the nasopharynx, below into the laryngeal pharynx, and anteriorly to the mouth. The fauces separate the oropharynx from the mouth and consist of the soft palate and uvula above, and two folds on either side extending from the soft palate to the tongue, called the anterior and posterior pillars of the fauces. The faucial tonsils lie between the anterior and posterior pillars.

The **Laryngeal Pharynx** runs from the level of the epiglottis to the lower border of the cricoid cartilage. Its anterior wall presents from above down towards the inlet to the larynx, the posterior surface of the arytenoid cartilages and of the cricoid cartilages. Behind this, the pharynx leads into the œsophagus.

ANATOMY OF THE PHARYNX

The pharynx as a whole is a muscular tube without a front wall and is a potential space only. Its muscles originate in the side walls of the nose, mouth and larynx, and meet behind, in front of the 2nd to the 6th cervical vertebræ. These muscles are in three groups: the superior, middle and inferior constrictors, and they contract during swallowing and push the food on. They are supplied by branches of the vagus nerve. The

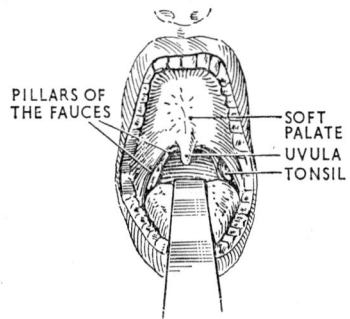

Fig 24.—Looking into the Mouth with the Tongue Depressed.

glossopharyngeal nerve (9th cranial nerve) supplies the mucous membrane of the pharynx with sensory branches.

The Lymphoid Tissue of the Pharynx.—There are superficial masses of the lymphoid tissue in the pharyngeal mucosa which form a ring acting as a filter protecting the body against infecting organisms that might enter it from the nose or mouth. This ring of lymphoid tissue, "Waldeyer's ring" (Fig. 25), consists of the *faucial or palatine tonsils*, the *pharyngeal tonsil*, the *lingual tonsil* (which lies at the back of the tongue, immediately above the epiglottis) and scattered *lymphoid nodules* occurring on the posterior and lateral walls of the pharynx. This tissue appears to aid in the production of immunity, for it increases normally during childhood, when immunity is being acquired. Except in the presence of chronic infection, the pharyngeal lymphoid tissue begins to atrophy at about the time of puberty.

The pharyngeal tonsil lies on the roof and upper posterior wall of the nasopharynx. It contains many tubular crypts extending from the surface. Its surface has five or more fissures running from before backwards, the lymphoid follicles being arranged along the

FIG. 25.—WALDEYER'S RING OF LYMPHOID TISSUE.

sides of these fissures and crypts. There is no defined fibrous tissue capsule separating the pharyngeal tonsil from the superior constrictor muscle, so that complete surgical removal of all lymphoid tissue is not possible during adenoidectomy, and regrowth frequently occurs.

The faucial tonsils consist of lymphoid tissue with 8 to 20 tubular crypts which frequently branch in the depth of the tonsil. Whereas the adenoid is covered with ciliated mucous membrane which keeps the fissures swept clean of debris, the faucial tonsil is covered with stratified squamous epithelium, and desquamated epithelial cells and lymphocytes normally collect in the crypts. The faucial tonsil is enclosed in a capsule which

ANATOMY OF THE PHARYNX

enables complete enucleation of all tonsillar material by splitting the capsule.

The lymphatics of the pharynx are numerous, and drain into the anterior cervical glands, in front of the

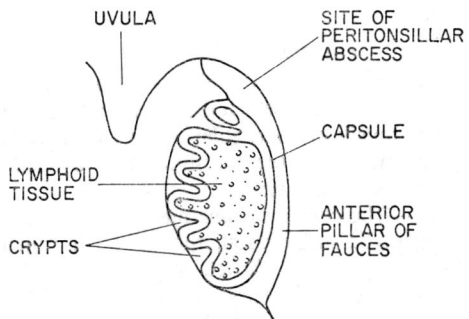

Fig. 26.—The Faucial Tonsil.

sternomastoid muscle, except those from the nasopharynx and posterior oropharynx, some of which drain into the posterior cervical lymph glands, behind the same muscle.

12

Diseases of the throat

Acute Inflammations

Acute inflammation of the throat is a distressingly common condition, of which the chief symptom is soreness. The tonsils are particularly likely to be involved in the infection and the tonsillitis then overshadows the adjacent inflammation.

Causes.—The causes of inflammation are:

1. Hæmolytic streptococci, though other organisms usually found in the throat, such as *Streptococcus viridans*, pneumococci, Neisseria catarrhalis, and viruses, may be increased in such infection.
2. Staphylococci, especially in the summer.
3. Corynebacterium diphtheriae.
4. Vincent's infection—an association of a spirillum and a fusiform bacillus.
5. Thrush, caused by *Candida albicans*.
6. Syphilis.
7. Blood diseases, such as acute leukæmia and agranulocytic angina.

Streptococcal Sore Throat (Acute Follicular Tonsillitis)

Signs and Symptoms.—This infection is abrupt in onset and usually occurs when the victim's resistance is lowered by fatigue, chilling, or coryza. The inflammation is concentrated in the faucial tonsils and penetrates deeply into the mucous membrane. On inspection, the uvula is seen to be inflamed and thickened, the tonsils are red and swollen and there are spots of yellowish exudate from the tonsillar crypts. The anterior cervical glands, below the angle of the jaw, are enlarged

DISEASES OF THE THROAT

and tender. There may be continuous pain at the back of the throat, with a sensation of rawness, or the patient may complain of severe pain only on swallowing. The temperature rises sharply to 39°C (102°F), or higher, and the initial rise may be accompanied by rigor.

In the course of a severe infection, ulceration of the tonsil surface occurs, and patches of exudate form a membrane which is distinguishable from diphtheria in that it can be detached. Diagnosis is confirmed by culture from a throat swab.

Complications.—Occasionally, ulceration in the depths of the crypts leads to the formation of thrombi in the vessels at the base of the tonsils. This results in systemic infections such as acute nephritis, arthritis and rheumatic fever, with or without cardiac involvement. Symptoms of these complications appear after the sore throat and pyrexia have abated. If nephritis develops, albuminuria is found in the third week from the onset of the tonsillitis. Other complications that are liable to follow acute follicular tonsillitis, especially in the young, are extensions of the inflammation upward, or to the ears, or downward to the larynx. Œdema may be so great as to obstruct respiration and swallowing.

Treatment.—Acute streptococcal tonsillitis is generally a self-limiting disease and will subside in a few days.

The patient should be confined to bed and isolated to prevent droplet infection. Hot gargles of normal saline, sodium bicarbonate or other mild lotion may be used, but as the effort of gargling sometimes increases the pain, and the lotion does not reach the whole of the inflamed area, treatment by throat spray with a sulpha drug or antibiotic as indicated by sensitivity test on throat swab is generally preferred. The sucking of lozenges keeps up the salivary secretion and tends to prevent stiffness of the neck muscles. Many varieties of lozenge dispensed for this purpose contain such drugs as phenol and ammonium bromide.

Applications of hot flannel or wool held in position by a figure-of-eight bandage round the neck and axillæ will act as a splint to a swollen aching throat and will give a surprising amount of relief. Four-hourly steam inhalations with menthol or tincture of benzoin compound are commonly ordered.

The diet is necessarily fluid at the onset of tonsillitis, when the temperature is high, swallowing difficult and the throat raw. It may be difficult to persuade the patient to drink sufficiently, but he must be encouraged to take from 4 to 5 litres daily. Lemon drink, orangeade and barley water are generally much appreciated and should be alternated with milk variously flavoured. Fluids can be made highly nourishing by the addition of glucose, lactose, Ovaltine, malted milk, chocolate, or beaten egg, according to the patient's taste. The doctor may order additional vitamins. As soon as the patient is capable of taking more substantial food, his appetite should be tempted. A child may be helped in swallowing if the nurse supports his neck with her hands as he makes the effort. Ice cream is often acceptable and soft solids may be swallowed more easily than liquids.

Frequent mouth-washes are necessary and should be used after every milk drink. Since the patient is confined to bed whilst fever is present, pressure areas require regular treatment and a daily blanket bath should be given at this stage. The bedclothes should be light and applied according to the patient's comfort.

A four-hourly temperature record should be kept, the urine tested daily, and the fluid intake and output measured.

Chemotherapy is the rule, and with it, the inflammation usually dies down after 4 or 5 days. The patient is toxæmic, if not septicæmic, and after an

DISEASES OF THE THROAT

acute attack of tonsillitis, suffers from weakness and fatigue for a few weeks. The chief principles to observe in order to lessen this debility are rest and nourishment. The patient is best kept in bed for several days after the temperature has returned to normal. An iron preparation (notably after haemolytic streptococcal infection) may be ordered, and a holiday is of great benefit.

Watch should be kept for systemic complications (see page 109). The first signs of acute nephritis are early morning œdema of the face, backs of the hands or ankles, and a diminished urinary output with albuminuria.

Any return of fever or complaint of pain in the joints should be reported to the doctor.

Acute Pharyngitis caused by hæmolytic streptococci in patients who have had the tonsils removed is seldom as severe an inflammation as that of acute follicular tonsillitis, but follows a similar course and may have the same complications. The inflammation begins in the nasopharynx and travels to the laryngeal pharynx or vice versa. The mucous membrane shows varying degrees of redness, and in the areas where tonsils have been removed, bright patches of lymphoid tissue are often seen. Exudate from these may become membranous as in tonsillitis and other signs and symptoms are similar.

Treatment follows the same lines as for tonsillitis, although the patient is not usually acutely ill and the temperature is only mildly raised.

Recurrent attacks of acute pharyngitis need investigation. It may be that there is an infective focus such as adenoids, infected tonsils, or tonsils incompletely removed. There may be allergy. Epidemics of pharyngitis due to milk are uncommon since the widespread use of pasteurisation.

Scarlet Fever (Scarlatina)

This is an acute pharyngitis or tonsillitis accompanied by a skin rash. The cause is a hæmolytic streptococcus of a special type which produces a toxin capable of causing the rash, though no rash occurs if the patient is already immune to the specific toxin. Many authorities therefore consider scarlet fever and acute tonsillitis as one and the same disease. Both types are equally infectious, and a victim of acute follicular tonsillitis may be much more ill than one with an extensive scarlet rash. However, scarlet fever is a notifiable disease, and the patient is nursed in isolation.

As scarlet fever is more common in childhood, before immunity is great, local complications such as otitis media, sinusitis and suppurative adenitis of the neck may occur as well as systemic infection. Fortunately the incidence of scarlet fever is decreasing.

Peritonsillar Abscess—"Quinsy"

This is an abscess in the cellular tissue outside the tonsil capsule, between it and the constrictor muscles of the pharynx. After repeated attacks of tonsillitis, an intra-tonsillar abscess in the depths of a stenosed crypt bursts laterally through the tonsil capsule.

Signs and Symptoms.—After a few days of tonsillitis, there is increasing pain on one side and increasing difficulty of swallowing. The patient holds his head stiffly towards the side of the abscess and is obviously in distressing pain. The throat is red, there is marked swelling of the soft palate on the side of the abscess, with displacement of the uvula to the opposite side. The tonsil itself is displaced toward the midline (see Fig. 27, also Fig. 26). The glands below the angle of the jaw are enlarged and tender but there is usually not much fever.

Complications most to be feared are a downward spread of the infection, œdema of the glottis and

DISEASES OF THE THROAT

thrombophlebitis of one of the large veins in the neck.

Treatment.—In addition to the treatment of the preceding tonsillitis, the patient should be provided with a sputum mug as he is unable to swallow his saliva.

When a rounded bulge indicates that the accumulated pus has become localized, the abscess is incised and drained, generally under a local anæsthetic. Penicillin therapy is usually continued until the inflammation has

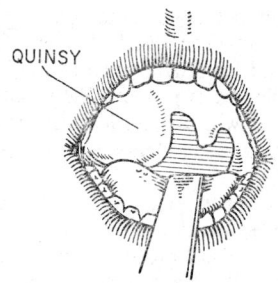

FIG. 27.—"QUINSY" OR PERITONSILLAR ABSCESS.

subsided completely. At this stage, whilst the patient's immunity is still high and before scar tissue has become dense, tonsillectomy is generally performed. Otherwise a recurrence of the quinsy is highly probable.

Retropharyngeal Abscess

This is a collection of pus between the posterior pharyngeal wall and the vertebræ. There are two types of abscess, acute and chronic.

1. **The Acute Form** is due to an infection in lymph glands situated one each side of the pharynx, superficial to the prevertebral fascia. These glands atrophy early in childhood, and therefore a retropharyngeal abscess of this type occurs only in infancy. The suppuration is usually one-sided.

Symptoms of Acute Retropharyngeal Abscess.—The illness may follow an upper respiratory infection such as coryza or measles. The degree of fever is variable. The chief symptom is difficulty of swallowing. The child refuses to feed or the food is regurgitated. As the abscess spreads downward, dyspnœa and inspiratory stridor develop owing to the narrowing of the airway. The child is extremely ill—restless, sweating, cyanosed and sometimes vomiting—and unless prompt treatment is instituted, the case ends fatally. An X-ray film of the neck helps the diagnosis.

Complications.—The chief dangers are respiratory obstruction and hæmorrhage from the internal carotid artery. If dyspnœa is present, the mouth must not be forcibly opened with a gag, lest this should cause the abscess to rupture suddenly and the septic material to be inhaled.

Treatment.—When diagnosis of retropharyngeal abscess is made, suction apparatus should be immediately procured. The abscess is incised, using as a rule a guarded scalpel. This procedure is usually carried out without anæsthetic with the child firmly wrapped in a blanket, lying on his back, with his head low. Then, as pus appears, he is turned quickly on to his abdomen, with head and shoulders over the edge of the table. Suction should be used as required. Tracheotomy instruments are kept at hand during and after the operation. Recovery is generally rapid. The incision should be kept open daily by the insertion of artery forceps until no more pus escapes.

Hæmorrhage from the carotid artery requires prompt ligation of the artery to avoid a recurrence. A child usually recovers from a first hæmorrhage but seldom survives a second. At the first warning—a few spots of blood coughed up—the nurse should immediately inform the surgeon.

2. **The Chronic Form** of retropharyngeal abscess is

due to tuberculosis of the bodies of the cervical vertebræ and occurs in older children and adults. The abscess causes bulging, often bilateral, of the posterior pharyngeal wall.

Both types of abscess are extremely dangerous. The head is held stiffly and there are violent pains especially at night. The abscess is opened through an external incision behind the sternomastoid muscle.

Faucial Diphtheria

Where immunization in infancy and childhood is universal, the disease has been almost completely wiped out. Such cases as occur in immunized persons are comparatively mild, and the early administration of antitoxin prevents the serious complications.

Course and Signs of the Disease.—An infection of the throat by the Corynebacterium diphtheriae is likely to be a much more serious condition than the nasal diphtheria described in an earlier chapter. It is transmitted in the same way—that is, by direct contact or from carriers harbouring the bacilli in the pharynx. The organisms settle in the tonsil and produce a toxin which destroys the surface epithelium. This causes an exudate of serum which coagulates and forms a dirty grey membrane—like the surface of a cut raw potato which has been left dry. The membrane is adherent and has well-defined margins. It spreads from the tonsils to the soft palate and sometimes on to the posterior pharyngeal wall. There is a "mousy" odour to the breath. The cervical lymph glands are enlarged and tender.

The incubation period is from 2 to 5 days. There is a gradual onset of sore throat, low-grade fever ($37 \cdot 5°–38°C$, $99°–101°F$) with an increase of pulse rate out of proportion to the rise in temperature. The pulse rate is frequently 120 to 140 beats per minute. Toxæmia is marked and the patient is very ill indeed although neither pyrexia nor sore throat are extreme. The tonsils are at first swollen and red; then the membrane appears. Speech is painful and has a nasal "twang", the patient talking as though he held a plum in his mouth. Diagnosis is confirmed by culture from a throat swab which has been rubbed over the membrane and then on to Loeffler's medium. It is examined after 12 to 18 hours.

Complications.—The complications that are likely to arise are due either to spread of the inflammation into the larynx, or to the spread of the toxins. While the bacilli remain in the local area they have invaded, the toxins produced spread through the lymphatic and blood circulation to the tissues. These toxins specifically affect the heart muscle and the nervous system causing myocardial damage and paralyses of various muscles, as for example, the soft palate, the eye muscles, the pharyngeal muscles and the diaphragm. Heart failure is the most usual cause of death from diphtheria due to degeneration of the cardiac muscle. The most common of the paralyses is that of the soft palate, which develops in the second or third week of the disease, after the acute symptoms have subsided, and lasts 2 or 3 weeks. It causes regurgitation of fluid through the nose. Paralysis of the eye muscles will cause squinting—this too disappears in a few weeks.

Œdema of the throat and membranous obstruction may require tracheostomy (see page 160).

Fortunately, the complications of diphtheria are seldom seen nowadays.

Treatment.—If diphtheria is suspected 20 to 40 thousand units of antitoxin are given immediately without waiting for the report on the throat swab. The patient should be put to bed and isolated—usually in an isolation hospital. The nursing treatment is carried out under strict isolation precautions. The nurse should be immune to diphtheria and should wear a mask and gown. The patient is nursed in the recumbent position, pillows being allowed only by the doctor's orders. He

DISEASES OF THE THROAT 117

is kept at complete rest, being fed and washed by the nurse until all danger of heart complications is past. Food is at first restricted to milky fluids, and semi-solids, since condiments and acid drinks such as lemonade are painful to swallow whilst the throat is raw. Thickened milk foods, such as cornflour, egg nog and custard are easily swallowed. Reaction to the large doses of antitoxin, or "serum sickness" should be watched for. This may give rise to fever, an urticarial rash, joint pains, and is treated symptomatically. It usually occurs 1 or 2 days after the injection. Rarely, anaphylactic shock occurs with the injection of antitoxin.

Glandular Fever—Infectious Mononucleosis

This is an infectious disease, the causative organism of which is a virus; the incubation period is 7 days. Its characteristic features are fever, enlargement of the lymphatic glands, including the tonsils, and changes in the blood. The white blood count is raised, the lymphocytes being especially increased, larger than normal and bluish. The Paul-Bunnel agglutination test is positive.

Signs and Symptoms.—The symptoms are malaise, headache and an unusually persistent sore throat. The cervical glands are especially affected, particularly those deep to the sternomastoid muscle, and may swell rapidly. Axillary glands are generally enlarged also. The tonsils, although red and swollen, do not produce an exudate except in those subject to tonsillitis.

Treatment.—The treatment is symptomatic. Recurrences occasionally extend over several weeks, and debility may persist for many months, but recovery is the rule.

Vincent's Angina

This is a specific infection of the mouth or pharynx due to the associated existence of a spirillum, and a fusiform bacillus. The disease may occur in epidemics, being transmitted by direct contact, or frequently arises from organisms already existing in the mouth when there is lack of oral hygiene or of vitamin C.

Signs and Symptoms.—The first sign is a dirty-grey, punched-out ulcer usually on one tonsil. The ulceration spreads over the gums, there is soreness of throat and mouth, slight pyrexia and enlargement of the cervical glands. Sloughs form at the bottom of the ulcers, covering granulations that bleed easily. The odour of the breath is particularly offensive. The diagnosis is supported by finding fusiform bacilli and spirilla in large numbers in a smear from an ulcer.

Treatment.—The patient is not usually kept in bed, nor is he isolated except for keeping separate his feeding utensils. As full a diet is given as can be taken with comfort, and large amounts of vitamin C—for example: 200 milligrams of ascorbic acid twice daily. Intramuscular injection of penicillin usually brings about recovery in 36 hours. Intravenous neoarsphenamine and similar preparations of arsenic have been used, the first dose of 0.3–0.45 grammes being repeated after 48 hours. The local treatment consists of mouth-washes after every meal or drink, and thorough cleansing of the teeth. If a tooth-brush is used, it should be a soft one and, when not in use, should be kept in an antiseptic solution, such as sodium hypochlorite.

The patient should be examined by the doctor 4 days after the pyrexia and adenitis have subsided. Frequently, dental treatment is deemed necessary.

Another method of treating Vincent's angina is to paint the affected area with 5 per cent. neoarsphenamine in glycerin and then to insufflate with bismuth subnitrate powder four times a day. Since the condition is very common and is often difficult to cure, the nurse may meet a variety of treatments with different patients and different surgeons.

Fungal Stomatitis ("Thrush")

Thrush is stomatitis (inflammation of the mouth) or pharyngitis characterized by adherent small white patches on the mucous membrane. It is due to a fungus, commonly *Candida albicans*. Very little inflammation occurs under the patches and there are often no other symptoms—no sore throat or fever—except loss of taste and appetite. It occurs in infants on the cheeks and lips, and in adults (generally those on a milk diet) on the faucial and lingual tonsils and on the pharyngeal lymph nodes. The condition is usually considered due to neglect of oral hygiene and in the sterilization of infant feeding bottles and teats. It seldom arises in breast-fed babies.

Treatment.—The treatment consists of gentle cleaning of the mouth in an adult—a 1 or 2 per cent. aqueous solution of gentian violet may be painted over the patches every few days. A nystatin suspension or lozenges may be used. For a baby, the self-cleansing by a teaspoonful of boiled water after feeds is the only local treatment. The feeding bottles should be kept scrupulously clean. After washing, they should be boiled or immersed in a solution of sodium hypochlorite.

Syphilis of the Throat

Primary syphilis—chancre of the tonsil—is extremely rare. One or two cases have been reported and have been ascribed to the use of a contaminated drinking vessel. An indurated swelling occurs, with ulceration and a sore throat which persists longer than a week. Diagnosis is made by finding the organism, the *Treponema pallidum*, in a swab taken from the ulcer.

Secondary syphilis frequently causes a sore throat, some 6 to 12 weeks after primary infection. The mucous membrane shows dull red areas, slightly elevated on which are round, oval or long patches of ulceration with defined borders and a shining, pearly surface ("snail-track" ulcers). These usually occur on the tonsils or pillars of the fauces or on the inner surface of the lips. They are accompanied by moderate, remittent pyrexia, generalized enlargement and hardness of lymph glands, and skin rashes. The organisms can be demonstrated in the blood stream, the Wassermann reaction is strongly positive and the patient at this stage is highly infectious.

Treatment.—Specific anti-syphilitic treatment is necessary. Modern methods rely on penicillin or streptomycin therapy, older ones on the injection of bismuth.

The nursing treatment consists largely of preventing the spread of infection. This can occur only by inoculation, but any abrasion of the skin or mucous membrane might allow the organisms to enter. The patient's feeding and washing utensils should be kept separate and the nurse should wear gloves when attending him.

Agranulocytic Angina

Cause.—This sore throat is due to damage of the bone marrow by infection or drugs, especially by amidopyrine, gold, thyroid-suppressing drugs, some steroids, some antibiotics (particularly chloramphenicol) and sulphonamides. The agranulocytosis is more frequent when large doses of the drug are given over a long period, or when the patient has been sensitized by previous administration (see page 43).

Symptoms.

1. The patient suffers from marked prostration.

2. Rapidly spreading ulceration occurs on the tonsils, pharynx and mouth, with pain.

3. A white blood count, which is diagnostic, shows a diminution or absence of polymorphonuclear leucocytes. The total white cell count is low—for example, 2,000 per cubic millimetre of blood.

4. Fever is slight in mild cases, severe in acute ones.

5. Jaundice may occur, or cyanosis in sulphonamide poisoning.

6. Hæmorrhage sometimes arises from the ulcers.

7. Death may occur within a few days from the onset of the ulceration.

Treatment.—The drug responsible for the condition must be discontinued. Intravenous injection of 1 or 2 grammes of pentose nucleotide may be given daily to stimulate the bone marrow, or intramuscular injection of 10 ml of an 8 per cent. solution twice daily. Large doses of penicillin and transfusion of fresh blood may be given. In successful cases, the leucocyte count begins to return to normal about 5 days after the treatment commences. Instramuscular injections of BAL (British Anti-Lewisite) have also been given as treatment of metallic poisons.

Local treatment of the sore throat is required—in particular, irrigation and anæsthetic lozenges.

Acute Leukæmia

In acute leukæmia there is a permanent increase in the number of white blood cells. These excess cells are abnormal and have no protective function. The cause is the subject of much research.

The tonsils may be red, swollen and ulcerated. The glands are generally enlarged. There is sore throat, fever, hæmorrhage from the mucous membranes, and a rapidly progressive anæmia.

The treatment is symptomatic as there is no known cure at present.

Chronic Diseases of the Pharynx

Chronic Tonsillitis

This usually follows an acute attack of tonsillitis caused by hæmolytic streptococci.

Signs.—The tonsils and the anterior pillars of the fauces are persistently reddened. The tonsils may be enlarged or may be small and fibrous, and in their crypts collects an abnormal amount of caseous debris. Ulceration occurs in the depths of the crypts and liquid pus can generally be expressed from them on slight pressure from a spatula. Sometimes the crypts are sealed off, and then small abscesses result.

Local Symptoms.—These include mild soreness with recurrent attacks of acute inflammation, an unpleasant-tasting exudate from the tonsils and discomfort located in the cervical glands.

General Symptoms.—Loss of appetite, chronic fatigue, acute and chronic arthritis, fibrositis, neuritis, iritis and other subacute infections occur for which the diseased tonsils act as a focus.

The only satisfactory treatment is tonsillectomy.

Adenoids

The pharyngeal tonsil normally reaches its maximum development in mid-childhood, then atrophies and disappears at puberty. With chronic infection, enlargement of the tissue, called "adenoids" occurs, and frequently persists into adult life. (For "adenoid facies" see Chapter 3 and Fig. 3.)

Symptoms.—The *local symptoms* are due to nasal obstruction and are mouth-breathing, snoring, and frequent, prolonged head colds. These lead to sinusitis with a typical copious nasal discharge; or recurrent or chronic suppurative otitis media when the Eustachian tubes are infected. Defective hearing may become permanent deafness due to blockage of the tubes.

The *general symptoms* are the same as for chronic tonsillitis.

Treatment.—This is at first conservative, by correction of diet, plenty of fresh air and exercise and by breathing exercises. Should the adenoid tissue enlarge to reach the upper level of the posterior nares, adenoidectomy is performed. In most cases, all symptoms then disappear spontaneously, and children improve both in appearance and in mental capacity.

Hyperplasia of lymphoid tissue in children may be treated with small doses of deep X-ray when the condition has not been relieved by adenoidectomy or has recurred.

Chronic Pharyngitis

A chronic inflammation of the pharynx, without the formation of ulcers may result from allergy, alcohol or smoking, or be an extension of atrophic rhinitis or sinusitis, or accompany metabolic diseases such as anæmia, diabetes, gout.

Signs.—The signs are a diffuse redness, the enlargement of superficial lymph nodules, dryness of the throat and sometimes crusting, especially of the nasopharynx. There is a sense of irritation, soreness at times, with slight discomfort on swallowing.

Treatment.—The treatment is directed towards the general health, and the cause is removed if known. Smoking should be avoided.

Tuberculous Pharyngitis

This condition is secondary to pulmonary tuberculosis. Irregular, shallow ulcers with pale granulations can be seen in the pharynx and there is pain on swallowing. Signs of general tuberculosis, such as fatigue, wasting and evening pyrexia are present. Treatment of the lung condition must be instituted, and with its improvement, the pharyngitis clears up.

Syphilitic Pharyngitis

With tertiary syphilis, gumma may appear in the pharynx, causing, as elsewhere, painless swellings, with a tendency to ulcerate and to heal with much scarring.

Perforations of the palate or of the faucial pillars may result.

General treatment of syphilis is required, local applications having little effect.

Actinomycosis

This disease is caused by the "ray fungus", a vegetable parasite which occasionally attacks the pharynx. It causes a firm, painless swelling which proceeds to ulceration and suppuration, the discharge containing the distinctive yellow "sulphur granules".

Treatment.—The treatment is to give iodides internally, Lugol's iodine being frequently prescribed. A prolonged course of penicillin has also proved effective.

New Growths of the Pharynx

Benign New Growths

A *papilloma* most often grows from the base of the uvula and is pedunculated.

An *adenoma* is rare. It occurs in the uvula or soft palate and forms a firm swelling under the mucous membrane.

A *fibroma* occurs as a rounded growth, most often on the posterior pharyngeal wall.

All the above tumours can be removed surgically.

Hæmangiomata are sometimes found on the posterior pharyngeal wall. They are bluish, and may be sessile or pedunculated. They bleed easily when touched. The treatment is by cauterization or by radiotherapy.

Malignant New Growths

These rarely occur before forty years of age.

Carcinoma may involve any part, but chiefly the lower lateral pharyngeal wall.

Carcinoma and Sarcoma of the Tonsil

Both types of new growth of the tonsil occur. If a unilateral enlargement, which is inflamed, does not respond to local treatment, biopsy should be done. A malignant growth develops rapidly into an ulcer with a hard irregular edge. In early cases there is no enlargement of glands, but glands at the angle of the jaw are occasionally the first sign of the disease.

Symptoms.—The symptoms are proportionate to the extent of the lesion. If the pillars, the tongue and the posterior pharyngeal wall are involved, there is difficulty in swallowing. The movements of the tongue are restricted. The patient complains of pain radiating to the ear. Later, excessive mucus occurs, occasionally some bleeding, and more pain. When the new growth is confined to the tonsil, the prognosis is good.

Treatment.—Radiotherapy is particularly successful in this type of malignancy, but radical dissection of secondarily invaded glands may be needed.

Carcinoma of the Lower Pharynx

This usually occurs behind the cricoid cartilage in women or in the piriform fossa in men (see page 138). It is a firm, elevated growth which breaks down in the centre, leaving an ulcerated area with a crater-like indurated rim.

Symptoms.—The symptoms vary from a vague discomfort, such as a sensation of fulness to pain extending to the ear. There is rapid invasion of the adjacent tissue and glands, so that an early diagnosis is imperative for cure.

Treatment.—Piriform fossa lesions do reasonably well on radiotherapy, but the glands usually need surgery. Post-cricoid cases are rarely affected by radiotherapy and radical surgery provides the only hope.

Growths of the nasopharynx are rare but occasionally the Eustachian tube may be blocked by a growth.

Radiotherapy or the insertion of radium is usually indicated. An operation has been devised in which a transpalatal incision is made where the soft palate joins the hard palate. The soft palate then drops down and the nasopharynx can be explored, in order to establish a diagnosis or to remove a benign tumour.

13

Tonsillectomy and adenoidectomy

In childhood, these two operations for removal of tonsils and adenoids are commonly performed together as treatment for chronic inflammation. In adult life, tonsillectomy is frequently all that is needed, the adenoids having atrophied. The operation usually takes place a few weeks after the occurrence of sore throat. It is contra-indicated in the presence of an acute infection (especially of the respiratory tract) or blood disease such as hæmophilia or anæmia. The patient is admitted to hospital at least 1 day before operation.

The two chief methods of removing tonsils are:

Enucleation of the Tonsils by Dissection.—This is essential for long-standing inflammation and after peritonsillar abscess.

Enucleation by Guillotine.—This operation is a rapid one and very satisfactory in skilled hands. It is particularly popular when there are large numbers of patients to be treated.

Preparation of a Child for Hospital Treatment

The psychological effect on a small child of a period in hospital depends a great deal upon the age and emotional development of the child and upon the preparation given by his parents before admission. The duration in hospital for tonsillectomy is short and the subjects are usually of the age to accept brief explanation of what is to be expected. Being a patient in hospital can be a valuable and is often an enjoyable experience, but children need preparation to face what is strange and unpleasant. Parents can be given guidance on how to help their children and frequently need reassurance themselves. Many hospitals issue leaflets of information and advice to parents of children awaiting admission and sometimes a separate welcoming leaflet is given to the child himself. A recent research has shown that most school children whose views were asked had fear of operations and anæsthetics. Some of those who had been patients emphasized the fears they had had before operation rather than any post-operative experiences.

When possible, the mother should bring her child to the ward, help him undress and stay for as long as she is able. A young child should be allowed to keep a favourite toy or possession. There should be mutual understanding between parents and nursing staff and arrangements should be made for telephone enquiries, visiting and fetching the child home.

Pre-operative Treatment

The procedure following the admission of the patient follows the usual routine. The history of the patient is taken and the throat, heart and lungs are examined. The urine is tested and, if necessary, the bleeding and clotting times are estimated. Apart from attention to the cleanliness of the mouth and the removal of dentures if worn, no preparation of the throat is required. The meal before operation is omitted. Children are usually given a sedative such as Nembutal or Vallergan syrup an hour or more before operation and oral atropine, the dose varying according to the child's weight. Otherwise, premedication before general or local anæsthesia follows the preference of the anæsthetist.

A general anæsthetic is chosen for children, for nervous adults and those with adenoids. Local infiltration anæsthesia is an alternative, and many surgeons prefer this as it is considered that there is less bleeding and soreness and the patient makes a more rapid recovery than after a general anæsthetic.

Dissection of Tonsils

There are many methods of performing this operation and almost every throat specialist has his preferences regarding his own position, the patient's position, the instruments used and the technique followed. The main differences in procedure are: blunt dissection, using long-bladed dissecting forceps, and sharp dissection, using scissors. Some surgeons combine the two. The aim is to dissect the tonsil in the plane of its capsule and ensure that it is completely removed. The dissection is carried below the lower pole of the palatine tonsil, to exclude the lingual tonsil which extends along the base of the tongue. If diseased tonsil remnants are left, they are apt to cause further trouble. Even after a thorough tonsillectomy, lymphoid tissue occasionally enlarges and tonsillitis recurs.

Operation under General Anæsthesia

Some children are especially frightened when it comes to the moment of lying down to take the anæsthetic, but the terror disappears if they are allowed to sit up and watch the proceedings. Therefore a child if not already drowsy is sometimes allowed to sit up for the commencement of anæsthesia, then, as the fumes make him sleepy he is placed on his back. For an adult, the anæsthetic is given with the patient lying flat. The choice of anæsthetic depends upon the agreement of surgeon and anæsthetist. As soon as relaxation occurs, the patient's head is placed in the desired position for operation. If suction is used during operation, no aspiration of blood will occur. A mouth gag is inserted, of a type such as Davis's, with a small, medium or large tongue blade according to the size of the patient. The gag is opened, and to a metal tube on it is attached rubber tubing which connects with the vaporizer. The surgeon takes up his position and his head lamp is adjusted. The suction tube is placed ready at hand, and the instrument table on his left.

Some surgeons remove adenoids (if present) first, so that the bleeding from the nasopharynx shall have ceased before the patient returns to bed. With his gloved finger, the operator feels for the enlarged tissue behind the palate. Then, using a La Force adenotome or a guarded curette, the adenoids are gently swept off in one piece. A small gauze pack 25 mm by 38 mm, tied with a length of tape is inserted into the nasopharynx with the tape hanging out of the mouth and left until the completion of the operation.

For tonsillectomy, the tonsil is drawn forward by a volsellum or special tonsil-holding forceps, and then it is dissected from its bed. Frequent mopping or suction is required to keep the pharynx clear of blood. Bleeding points are picked up and ligated with linen thread. Suturing is rarely needed, but if so, the stitch should be removed the following day. Sometimes, each tonsil fossa is packed for a short time with a mop soaked in adrenaline solution. The post-nasal pack is removed and a final inspection is made to see that no gauze mops are left behind, and a count is made. The patient is then turned well over on his side. The coughing and swallowing reflexes may have returned before he leaves the theatre. If the cough reflex is not fully recovered, the patient is sent back to the ward with a gag in position. The handing over of responsibility from the anæsthetist to the nurse should be clearly stated.

Operation under Local Anæsthesia

The patient should be sitting upright. A sterile sheet should be placed over him and a basin on his knees held in both hands. He sucks a Nupercaine lozenge before going to the theatre or his throat may be sprayed before operation with cocaine 5 per cent.

Nupercaine 1 per cent. solution containing 0.3 ml of 1:1000 adrenaline to 30 ml is injected into the pillars. After waiting a few minutes, the surgeon grasps the tonsil and dissects it out.

Dissection is often almost bloodless, but if there are fibrous adhesions, sharp scissors are required and some bleeding may result. As under general anæsthesia, bleeding points are ligated.

Post-operative Treatment

As soon as the effect of the local anæsthetic wears off, the patient may need an injection of morphine 10 mg or pethidine 50 mg. Then codeine 30 mg and aspirin 600 mg may be given 4-hourly.

The Guillotine Operation

As soon as the child is under the anæsthetic, the mouth is opened widely with a gag such as Doyen's. A guillotine, for example Heath's or Ballenger's, is used, and the tonsil is pushed by the surgeon's finger through the ring of the guillotine, the blade is pushed home and the tonsil is peeled off by the surgeon's forefinger. If necessary, the adenoids are then removed with a curette and the patient is turned on his face so that the blood runs out of his mouth. Bleeding quickly ceases. The surgeon inspects the throat, the anæsthetist satisfies himself that the cough reflex has returned and the child is put back to bed in the position shown on page 102.

Post-operative Treatment

The immediate treatment after tonsillectomy has already been described on page 102. The outstanding aim is to maintain a clear airway and prevent asphyxia from inhaled blood and blood clots. Sips of water are allowed as soon as the patient is awake, and when vomiting has ceased, he is encouraged to swallow. This prevents stiffness of the pharyngeal muscles, and militates against infection. The more he swallows the easier it becomes. An aspirin mixture may be gargled and swallowed every few hours (for example, 20 minutes before meals). Children suffer comparatively little pain, and ice cream and jelly usually tempt them to swallow. A child is usually sent home the second day if the temperature is below 37.5°C (99°F), and there is no bleeding. Adults do not recover as rapidly and it is important that they should not become dehydrated by refusing to swallow. The morning after operation, a light diet is given, and thereafter the patient is encouraged to return to ordinary diet. A simple gargle of glycerin of thymol is given after meals. The patient is allowed out of bed on the day after operation and goes home in normal cases within the week.

Rarely, the throat is so painful that a spray of phenol 1 per cent, in warm water is used to irrigate the tonsil beds.

Complications after Tonsillectomy and Adenoidectomy

Hæmorrhage

This may be reactionary, occurring within 12 hours of operation, or secondary, 5 to 7 days afterwards. The latter is due to sepsis. For signs of post-operative bleeding see page 103. The surgeon should be informed. While waiting for him, the foot of the bed is raised and the patient's head kept in a dependent position.

Treatment of Bleeding from Tonsillar Fossæ

The surgeon removes the clot carefully by means of Luc's forceps. He then mops the fossa with wool soaked in hydrogen peroxide. If this does not cause the bleeding to stop, it may be necessary to take the patient back to the theatre and ligate one or more vessels.

Treatment of Bleeding from Adenoids

It is rarely necessary to assist nature in controlling bleeding after adenoidectomy, and sitting the child up may be all that is required, but if troublesome bleeding should occur it may be treated by inserting post-nasal packs. The surgeon may first retract the uvula in order to remove a tag of adenoid tissue.

FIG. 28.—POST-NASAL PACK READY FOR INTRODUCTION.

For the packs two strips of ribbon gauze folded and tied to a size of approximately 25 mm by 38 mm by tape or linen thread, or two marine sponges, are required. A soft rubber catheter is passed along the floor of one nostril until it appears in the pharynx. It is then pulled out through the mouth sufficiently far to enable the operator to tie one of the packs to the eye end.

A second thread is attached to the pack and brought out through the mouth for the removal of the pack in due course. The end of the catheter protruding from the nostril is then pulled back through the nose, bringing the thread with it until further withdrawal of the thread is prevented by the lodgement of the pack in the post-nasal space. The catheter is then detached. The threads are secured to the cheeks by small pieces of adhesive tape.

Fig. 29.—Post-nasal Pack in Position, with Tapes tied across Small Gauze Swab Anteriorly. Thread through Mouth not shown.

The packing is usually left for 24 hours and then removed by cutting the thread from the nose and withdrawing the pack by the thread through the mouth. Should bleeding recur, fresh packing will be inserted.

Since sepsis is likely to be present, penicillin "cover" is usually given to prevent infection going up the Eustachian tubes.

Atelectasis (Partial Collapse of Lung)

This complication may arise if a plug of mucus blocks one of the bronchial tubes. The signs are fever, rapid breathing, dyspnœa, cough and cyanosis. There will be dullness in the affected side with absence of breath sounds over the area involved. Radiographs will show that the heart is displaced toward, and the diaphragm is raised on, the collapsed side.

The treatment is to move the patient about. Breathing and coughing exercises are begun. He should sit in a chair if possible and cough. Carbon dioxide may be administered. If these measures fail, early bronchoscopy is performed in order to aspirate the occluding plug.

Pneumonia

At first the clinical picture of pneumonia is the same as that of atelectasis. Breath sounds, however, are increased and X-rays will show a different picture.

Lung Abscess

This complication is very rare if the head is hyperextended during operation, thus preventing inhalation of any material such as blood and mucus.

The signs are fever, cough and purulent sputum occurring 1 to 2 weeks after operation.

Discharge of a Child after Tonsillectomy

When the time comes for the child to go home, the mother is usually asked to come to the ward to dress him. She is advised that he will need extra rest for a few days but that normal food should be taken. If he should become at all feverish, the doctor should be consulted.

Special breathing exercises are sometimes recommended. These are usually taught in a physiotherapy clinic, for which the mother and child are given an appointment.

Breathing Exercises after Tonsillectomy and Adenoidectomy

The habit of nasal speech which a child develops from enlargement of the adenoids is difficult to eliminate without perseverance. Certain exercises have been devised before which the child should blow his nose, one nostril at a time. It is essential that the mouth should be kept shut during the exercises, of which the following are examples.

1. Breathe in deeply via the nose. Breathe out slowly.

2. The arms are raised above the head whilst breathing in, and lowered on expiration. The shoulders must not be raised and the arms should be well back to expand the chest.

3. Whilst the nurse or mother keeps a hand on the child's back he should take a deep breath through the nose and try to push the hand away, at the same time pulling in his abdomen. Then he should breathe out through the nose, relaxing the abdomen.

4. Humming through the nose is amusing and beneficial. The child may think of going up a steep hill whilst breathing in and pushing hard downhill when breathing out.

These exercises should be performed two or three times daily and initially are best done in groups.

Section IV: The Larynx, Trachea and Œsophagus

14

Anatomy of the larynx. Voice production. Swallowing

All animal life originally was aquatic and derived oxygen from water. Lungs were therefore unnecessary. As the water receded it was necessary for animals to take oxygen from the air instead of from water, and lungs gradually developed instead of gills. To protect the lungs from mud a closing valve was evolved. This was the origin of the larynx, which was concerned with respiration and not with the voice. Voice production developed incidentally, as the valve was used to retain air that had been inspired. To illustrate this, think of a frog suddenly disturbed on the bank of a pond. It gulps a supply of air with a snapping sound as it plunges into the water. The sound is not made when the frog enters the water without alarm or hurry—it is made partly by the closing of its mouth, partly by the closing of the valve-like orifice to its lungs. Through the ages, the simple form of larynx possessed by the lower vertebrates has evolved into a marvellous mechanism with many functions, culminating in those of speech and song.

The human larynx is made up of a more or less rigid framework of cartilages held together by ligaments and moved one on another by muscles. It is a box-like structure, approximately 38 mm in length, 32 mm in breadth and 25 mm in depth. It is lined with mucous membrane continuous with that of the pharynx above and of the trachea below. The larynx is separated from the 4th, 5th and 6th cervical vertebræ by the laryngeal portion of the pharynx, the anterior wall of which it forms. In this wall, on each side of the

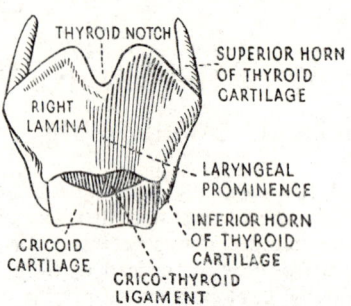

Fig. 30.—The Thyroid and Cricoid Cartilages (Anterior View).

larynx, is a recess known as the piriform fossa. The position of the larynx can be readily seen and felt in the front of the neck where it makes a variable pro-

Fig 31.—The Laryngeal Cartilages (Posterior View).

trusion—"Adam's apple" or the laryngeal prominence.

Laryngeal Cartilages.—The chief cartilages of the larynx are: the "shield-like" *thyroid cartilage* at the

ANATOMY OF THE LARYNX

front and sides; the "signet ring" *cricoid cartilage*, whose "ring" portion lies below the thyroid and whose "signet" closes the larynx behind; and the right and left *arytenoid cartilages* which are perched on the "signet". The relationship of these cartilages with each other is shown in Figs. 30 and 31: they articulate by small synovial joints.

In addition to the above cartilages, the *epiglottis* is important. It shares in the protective function of the larynx by covering the entrance to the larynx during the act of swallowing. The epiglottis is a leaf-shaped portion of cartilage, its stem attached to the posterior aspect of the thyroid cartilage at the junction of the two thyroid plates. It curves upwards behind the tongue and the hyoid bone and cannot move forwards. Small muscles from the arytenoid cartilages pass to the sides of the epiglottis. In swallowing, the arytenoid cartilages are pulled forward, the tongue presses the epiglottis over the narrowed orifice of the larynx, and food slides over the smooth mucous membrane into the œsophagus.

The cartilages of the larynx are attached to each other by sheets and bands of fibrous tissue containing many elastic fibres. The upper horns of the thyroid cartilage articulate indirectly with the hyoid bone. From this the larynx is suspended. The hyoid bone itself is slung from the jaw by thick muscle, and the tongue is attached to the posterior aspect of the hyoid. Other muscles attach the hyoid bone to the larynx.

Vocal Cords.—Across the cavity of the larynx, on either side, are folds of tissue called the vocal cords. There are two pairs of these, one called the superior or false cords, and the other called the true vocal cords. The false cords are protective folds of connective tissue passing from half-way up the anterior border of the arytenoid cartilages forward to reach the angle of union between the two laminæ of the thyroid cartilage. The true cords pass from the bases of the arytenoid cartilages to points just below the false cords. They are composed of elastic tissue and project further into the cavity of the larynx than do the false cords.

Fig. 32.—The Inlet of the Larynx under Different Conditions as seen with the Aid of a Laryngoscope. A, Ordinary quiet inspiration. B, Very deep inspiration. C, Vocalization, especially in singing high notes.

The word "glottis" means the true vocal cords and the space between them (the sound-producing structures).

ANATOMY OF THE LARYNX

The space depends upon the position of the arytenoid cartilages.

When at rest, the vocal cords are in the V position shown in Fig. 32A and no sound is produced. In deep breathing the cords are pulled apart as in Fig. 32B. In phonation the cords are adducted, the space between narrows and in full adduction becomes a mere chink. The muscles which swing the arytenoids out sideways are of the voluntary striated type, so that the tension on the cords can be varied at will. The shorter the cords, the more rapid is their vibration as air passes through the glottis, and the higher is the pitch. In producing a "falsetto" voice, the glottis is much narrowed, as shown in Fig. 32C. During speech the cords are parallel to each other. The male larynx is larger than the female—the vocal cords are longer and this makes a man's voice deeper. The "breaking" of a boy's voice at puberty is due to growth changes in the larynx.

Nerves.—The nerve supply of the larynx is from:

1. The superior laryngeal branch of the vagus nerve, with external and internal branches. The internal branch pierces the thyrohyoid membrane and passes to the mucous membrane above the level of the cords. The external branch supplies the crico-thyroid muscle only.

2. The recurrent, or inferior laryngeal branch of the vagus nerve, passing to the other intrinsic muscles of the larynx.

Blood Vessels.—The arteries to the larynx are the superior laryngeal, from the external carotid artery, and the inferior laryngeal artery, from a branch of the subclavian artery.

The veins from the larynx enter either the internal jugular vein or the left innominate vein.

Swallowing

The act of swallowing takes place in two stages. First

the food bolus is pushed by the tongue into the pharynx whilst the nasopharynx is shut off by the lifting of the soft palate and the contraction of the superior constrictor muscles of the pharynx. Then the larynx is pulled forcibly upwards and forwards. At this moment, the bolus of food passes backwards over the larynx into the œsophagus, which opens reflexly to receive it.

Fig. 33.—The Relations of the Œsophagus.

The portion of the pharynx which lies behind the larynx is normally closed, as the posterior wall of the larynx is closely applied to the vertebral column. The œsophagus is a thin-walled tube commencing at the level of the cricoid cartilage. It passes first downwards, backwards and slightly to the left, then behind the arch of the aorta and the left bronchus, then slightly forwards and left to the opening in the diaphragm (see Fig. 33). The lumen of the œsophagus shows 5 constrictions:

1. At its commencement, opposite the sixth cervical vertebra.

2. At the entrance to the thorax.

3. Where the aorta crosses it, opposite the fourth dorsal vertebra.

4. Where the left bronchus crosses it, opposite the fifth dorsal vertebra.

5. Where it passes through the diaphragm, opposite the tenth dorsal vertebra.

Normally, the food is forced by active peristalsis down the œsophagus as far as the diaphragmatic constriction, where its level usually rises and falls once or twice before it passes into the stomach. This is shown by X-ray examination before a fluorescent screen, the patient being given barium emulsion to swallow.

15

Diseases of the larynx

Hoarseness is the chief symptom of disease of the larynx. It is the rough grating quality of voice, with a lower pitch than is normal for the individual, due to impaired vibration of the cords in response to the air column in the trachea. Very many diseases give rise to hoarseness, and though it is common with a severe cold or cough, any persistent hoarseness should be investigated as it is frequently an early sign of serious disease.

Stridor is a harsh shrill sound occurring during respiration when there is partial obstruction of the larynx. In quiet breathing the vocal cords scarcely move, but when obstructed, they are moved forcibly up and down with respiration.

Acute Infectious Laryngitis in Adults

This may occur as an entity but is usually associated with upper respiratory infection. The larynx becomes red and roughened, with, at first, scanty secretion.

Symptoms.—These are hoarseness which ranges from frequent breaking when speaking is attempted to complete loss of voice; a paroxysmal ineffective cough; and aching pain in the larynx. The temperature may rise to about 38°C (100°F) for 1 or 2 days.

Complications.—In an adult, these are generally comparatively slight. Spread of inflammation, for example, into the trachea is not uncommon and pulmonary complications may follow if the laryngitis is not properly treated.

Treatment.—The voice should be rested and steam inhalations given. The accompanying general respiratory infection should be treated.

DISEASES OF THE LARYNX

Laryngitis occurs as a complication of many acute specific diseases, such as measles, scarlet fever, whooping cough, typhoid fever, influenza, and in such cases the patient is severely ill. Meanwhile, the larynx and throat are watched so that a low tracheostomy can be performed should there be signs of obstructive laryngeal dyspnœa.

Acute Laryngitis in Children (or Croup)

The larynx of a child is small in proportion to the development of other regions; and the submucous tissue is looser than in adult life. Therefore, laryngitis in childhood is liable to be a much more serious condition than that described above. Œdema of the tissues and narrowing of the glottis is liable to occur, so dyspnœa may follow in a very short space of time. The condition is sometimes called spasmodic laryngitis. The spasms are short in duration and may be relieved by hot applications over the larynx. Very rarely, the obstruction requires tracheostomy, and instruments for this purpose should be kept in readiness.

Œdematous laryngitis occurs in a number of conditions, both traumatic and infective and is described in greater detail on pages 148 and 155.

Acute Laryngo-Tracheo-Bronchitis in Children

This is a serious condition occurring during epidemics of respiratory diseases and thought to be due to a filter-passing virus. Its onset is sudden and it may show itself as a fulminating laryngitis. Secondary bacterial infection occurs rapidly, particularly with the *Hæmophilus influenzæ*. Not only do the larynx and air passages become swollen, but the thick secretions formed readily cause obstruction and may even produce crusts.

Treatment.—This is urgent and consists of giving the child massive doses of penicillin and putting him into a Croupaire tent or steam tent filled with Alevaire. Alevaire is a non-irritating, non-toxic detergent, and its use favours the liquefying of the thick, tenacious secretions.

The child is watched with great care. If the obstruction to the airway increases and the general condition deteriorates, a tracheostomy is needed. The nurse has a special responsibility in such cases and must report instantly any increased restlessness or rise in pulse rate. Tracheostomy should be undertaken before any chest recession or cyanosis occurs.

After a tracheostomy has been carried out, repeated bronchoscopy and suction may be needed in order to free the lower airways of secretions and crusts.

Diphtheria of the Larynx

Pharyngeal and nasal diphtheria have already been considered in earlier sections (see pages 80 and 115).

Laryngeal diphtheria (uncommon now, since the discovery of the use of antitoxin) is usually an extension of the disease in the pharynx, but may occur primarily in the larynx, especially in children. The attack may be severe, as the diagnosis is not made as early as in faucial diphtheria and therefore the injection of antitoxin is delayed.

Symptoms.—The disease processes are similar to those of pharyngeal diphtheria, but the loose submucous tissue of the larynx swells early, and causes a cough and spasmodic stridor—commonly called "croup". The stridor and dyspnœa become increasingly severe. The special odour of the breath and the systemic signs of the disease are the same as in other forms of diphtheria. The diagnosis is usually made by indirect laryngoscopy. In appearance, the larynx is red and swollen; later, patches of grey exudate with slight bleeding at the edges may be seen, and still later, a diphtheritic membrane.

Treatment.—Antitoxin is given without waiting for confirmation of the diagnosis from culture of the swab. To relieve obstructive dyspnœa, tracheostomy may be

DISEASES OF THE LARYNX

required. The general treatment of the disease is as described earlier.

Nocturnal Dyspnœa in Children

Attacks of dyspnœa at night are frequently causes of great alarm. They occur after a child has been asleep for an hour or more. The dyspnœa is inspiratory, and accompanied by stridor. It lasts for a short period, then normal breathing returns, often with vomiting of thick mucus. The causes may be:

(*a*) Inflammatory, for example influenza or the onset of diphtheria.

(*b*) Non-inflammatory, which may be physiological.

Non-inflammatory Nocturnal Dyspnœa

During sleep, mucous secretions which normally drain from the pharynx into the œsophagus occasionally overflow into the larynx. This causes a sharp cough reflex and the glottis snaps shut, giving rise to air hunger. An attempt at inspiration draws the secretions below the larynx. Violent coughing then expels the residual air, which causes further air hunger. By this time the child is thoroughly awake and frightened. Soon, however, the glottis opens in response to the pull of the laryngeal muscles, the intruding matter is expelled and the coughing subsides with a hoarse croak. The child falls asleep and is quite well in the morning.

Many children have an occasional attack of this kind. If there is enlargement of the tonsils and adenoids, the attacks are more frequent and severe owing to the increase of secretion and the diminished airway.

Stridor of the Newborn

This condition is thought to be due to muscular weakness or incoordination. The entrance to the larynx tends to collapse inwards during inspiration. The stridor may be relieved by putting the infant in the prone position, whilst keeping watch that the nose and mouth are not obstructed. The condition usually settles itself after a few months.

Laryngismus Stridulus

This is a condition of childhood, particularly between two and six years of age. It is usually associated with rickets and is due to lack of Vitamin D.

Symptoms.—Without previous symptoms, the child wakens after a few hours' sleep with a peculiar, hollow cough. The cough is quickly followed by a crowing inspiration, and then the typical inspiratory, obstructive laryngeal dyspnœa sets in. The child becomes cyanosed and staring in the struggle for air. Gradually the cough and distress lessens, the attack subsides after 1 or 2 hours and the child falls asleep.

Treatment.—Reassurance is important. The child should be supported gently, patted and soothed in an encouraging manner. If available, oxygen is the best treatment of the attack. The room air should be kept warm and moist. A steam kettle may be used. The general health should be attended to, and the diet should contain sufficient milk, fruit, and additional vitamins. Artificial sunlight is valuable.

The outlook is good as long as the lack of vitamin D is not allowed to recur.

Angioneurotic Œdema

This condition is one form of giant urticaria in which the subcutaneous tissues are involved as well as the skin. It is due to allergy, and there is a nervous system element in the vasomotor disturbances manifested. The œdema may develop rapidly in the course of a few minutes. It affects the eyelids, lips, tongue, and throat, causing an alarming sense of suffocation.

Symptoms.—A tickling sensation is followed quickly by dyspnœa and signs of obstruction. The voice is

DISEASES OF THE LARYNX

muffled and deep. The larynx is so swollen that when viewed in a laryngeal mirror, it appears as a shapeless, purplish mass. Diagnosis is usually easy because of the associated skin condition, or because the patient is known to have suffered from previous attacks.

Treatment.—Slow subcutaneous injection of 0.2–0.6 ml of adrenaline hydrochloride will usually relieve the condition. Tracheostomy is rarely necessary, but a sterile set of instruments should be ready.

Local treatment of the larynx is not advised.

Investigation of the cause should be made (see hay-fever, page 78). Patients subject to angioneurotic œdema should be taught to give themselves adrenaline as required.

Chronic Laryngitis

The causes of persistent inflammation of the larynx are many:

1. Repeated infections of the respiratory tract and damage caused by coughing.
2. Vocal abuse, e.g. too much shouting at sporting events, straining the voice in singing, or using the voice during an acute attack of laryngitis.
3. Constant exposure to dust, tobacco or other smoke and irritants.
4. Mouth breathing.
5. Systemic causes such as alcoholism which produces chronic vasodilation.
6. Tumours, benign and malignant.
7. Syphilis.
8. Tuberculosis of the larynx which is always secondary to pulmonary tuberculosis.

Signs.—Indirect laryngoscopy shows a patchy, rough redness of the mucosa, which elsewhere is dull pink or grey. A stringy secretion covers the cords. By direct laryngoscopy, the roughness of the mucous membrane is more conspicuous, and the vocal cords appear rounded and thickened. The voice is intermittently hoarse and rough, and the individual is constantly clearing his throat, especially before speech. Chronic laryngitis is so common that this "ahem" has become a common practice to attract attention at the beginning of a speech.

Symptoms.—The patient complains of hoarseness, particularly after a night's sleep or after using the voice all day. The throat aches and feels swollen. A tickling sensation causes a constant slight cough.

Before a diagnosis of "chronic laryngitis" is made the possibility of tuberculosis, syphilis, or a new growth must be excluded, generally by biopsy.

Treatment.—Search must be made for a focus of infection. This may be in the nose, the sinuses, the tonsils or the teeth. Other predisposing causes, such as smoking, alcohol, and dust should be eliminated. Local treatment is not very satisfactory apart from thorough oral hygiene. The patient should be advised to sleep on the side, using a low pillow. This prevents the pharyngeal secretions from trickling into the larynx. Change to a warm moist seaside climate is helpful and a change of occupation must often be seriously considered. Silence is the best treatment, and if this is observed, perfect recovery can occur.

Vocal Nodules

These are due to overworking the voice, particularly if inflammation is present. They appear as little white points on the edge of the vocal cords, always at the junction of the anterior with the middle third, where the cords hit each other in phonation. With rest, they disappear; otherwise, they enlarge and may reach the size of a small pea.

Symptoms.—These are hoarseness and periodic complete loss of voice which results from the dropping

DISEASES OF THE LARYNX

of the nodule below the cords, where it may be nipped.

Treatment.—For the smallest nodules the only treatment is rest of the voice. A large nodule, or one that is not resolving is removed with punch forceps.

Laryngeal Polypi

With hypertrophy of the mucous membrane of the larynx, a polypus may form, usually one only. The commonest attachment is to the under surface of the anterior portion of one cord, from which it hangs in the subglottic space. It may not be seen on examination unless the patient is told to cough, when it is blown up and appears above the cords.

Symptoms.—Periodic sudden loss of voice occurs with as sudden a return.

Treatment.—This is removal by punch forceps or snare under direct vision.

Tuberculosis of the Larynx

The larynx is never the seat of primary tuberculosis, but is always secondary to pulmonary tuberculosis. As the latter is becoming rarer, so tuberculosis of the larynx is very uncommon.

Symptoms.—At first, the only symptom of a tuberculous larynx is in the voice, which is weak and intermittently husky. Talking is painful. Later, the swelling, ulceration, and perichondritis of the arytenoid cartilage leads to fixation of the cricoarytenoid joint and the vocal cord. The voice becomes more weak and husky, there is difficulty in swallowing, stridor, cough with sputum, and pain (frequently extending to the ear). Dyspnœa is rare. The outlook depends upon the condition of the lungs.

Signs.—Lesions of varying activity may be seen, often on the posterior laryngeal wall, or the interarytenoid region and involving the cords. The ulcers are shallow and indolent. Later, nodules of granulation give an uneven "mouse-nibbled" appearance to the cords.

Treatment.—By the use of streptomycin and PAS, complete healing may be expected. From the nurses' point of view, the treatment is that of open tuberculosis, and she must take the appropriate personal precautions.

Syphilis of the Larynx

Primary syphilis does not attack the larynx, but most patients with *secondary syphilis* have some laryngeal involvement. There is some erythema and the vocal cords have a mottled appearance. Occasionally, "snail-track" ulcers are seen on the epiglottis or arytenoids. The only symptoms are hoarseness and a raw sensation, and the only local treatment is steam inhalations.

Tertiary syphilis often has serious effects:

1. Gummata occur on the epiglottis, arytenoid eminences and false cords. They are deep red or purple with sometimes a central yellow spot showing an area of softening.

2. Deep ulcers supervene on the gummata. The ulcer has a sharp punched-out edge, with a grey and sloughing base, and is surrounded by an area of congestion.

3. Gummatous perichondritis, chiefly of the thyroid cartilage leads to swelling inside the glottis.

4. During healing the larynx becomes distorted by scar tissue. There may be destruction of the epiglottis, union of the vocal cords, stenosis of the subglottis, ankylosis of the cricoarytenoid joint.

Symptoms correspond to the pathological condition. The patient has a harsh, raucous voice. Extensive ulceration may exist without pain or difficulty in swallowing. Stenosis leads to stridor and dyspnœa which is worse at night, but is so insidious in onset that the patient becomes accustomed to it.

DISEASES OF THE LARYNX

In diagnosis, tuberculosis and malignant disease must be excluded. As the Wassermann and Meinicke reactions are sometimes negative in syphilis of the larynx, a section of a doubtful ulcer is examined under a microscope.

Treatment.—Systemic injections of penicillin or of bismuth are given. Permanent tracheostomy may be necessary for stenosis, but it must be a low incision (see page 167), owing to the danger of contraction of scar tissue.

Paralysis of the Larynx

The muscles of the larynx are supplied by the recurrent laryngeal nerve. This nerve may be paralysed owing to:

(*a*) Central lesions in the brain stem, as in bulbar palsy and some cerebellar tumours.

(*b*) Lesions affecting the vagus nerve in the neck.

(*c*) Lesions affecting the nerve after it leaves the vagus.

The latter include:

1. Pressure caused by aortic aneurysm.

2. Pressure from carcinoma of the bronchus, œsophagus, enlarged thyroid or other glands.

3. Injury such as cut throat or during operation on the thyroid gland.

4. Toxic effects of diphtheria, influenza, typhoid fever, syphilis.

The muscles first and most often affected are the abductors of the vocal cords. Paralysis of the adductors is more often hysterical in origin. According to the degree of paralysis, whether unilateral or bilateral, partial or complete, so the symptoms vary.

Sensory paralysis arises from interference with the superior laryngeal nerve. It may be due to pressure or to toxic peripheral neuritis as in general paralysis of the insane and tabes dorsalis.

The symptoms are anæsthesia, resulting in choking fits due to food going "the wrong way".

Treatment.—Very often no treatment is necessary, as the larynx learns to compensate for its own deficiency. The cause of the paralysis is treated if possible. Tracheostomy or intubation may be necessary in bilateral paralysis, or a plastic operation on the larynx may be performed. Frequent laryngoscopic aspiration may be used for patients with tabes dorsalis.

Injuries of the Larynx

Cut Throat

If the larynx is opened in a cut throat, the inhalation of blood will probably produce pulmonary complications. Tracheostomy should be performed below the injury, the latter being packed, and if necessary, repaired.

Blow on the Larynx

This may cause fracture of the cartilage or extravasation of blood into the laryngeal tissues. Perichondritis occurs, and fixation of one or both vocal cords, which may become permanent.

Symptoms.—There is tenderness over one or more cartilage. Swelling of the perichondrium enlarges the outline of the larynx and may lead to obstruction. Blood-stained sputum may be expectorated, or blood may be seen in the larynx.

Treatment.—Unless urgent symptoms appear, no interference is required, but the patient should be kept under observation. If there is much hæmorrhage, it may be necessary to open the larynx and tie the bleeding point; obstruction may call for tracheostomy.

Acute Obstruction of the Larynx

Signs.—Laryngeal obstruction of sudden onset or rapid progress needs little diagnosis—the trouble is obvious to any onlooker. The patient, so often a child, is brought to hospital with extreme difficulty of inspiration, accompanied by stridor and an ashy-grey face. Adults may have a grey or bluish tinge to their pallor. The difficulty of breathing is practically always inspiratory for various mechanical reasons and is accompanied by an indrawing of the chest wall. Children are usually very restless from anoxæmia, and this restlessness results in fatigue and desire for sleep. Should the obstruction not be relieved, the child eventually becomes unconscious as respiration ceases. Death from asphyxia can be prevented if the patient comes under surgical care before the heart has ceased to beat. It usually ceases within 3 or 4 minutes after cessation of respiration.

The *causes* of laryngeal obstruction are trauma, foreign bodies and disease. The history may make diagnosis obvious. Enquiry should be made as to whether any toy or small object has disappeared. The severity of the *symptoms* of obstruction depends upon the rapidity of its onset. A patient with a slowly developing stenosis of the larynx will learn to breathe slowly and with the least possible exertion, whereas one with a sudden obstruction, frightened at the sense of suffocation, makes violent efforts to take in more air and these close the larynx. The more sudden and violent the inrush of air, the more quickly and tightly do the folds of the glottis close.

The first-aid treatment consists in calmly convincing the patient, if an older child or an adult and not unconscious, that he can get more air if he does not try so hard to breathe in, and then in removing the obstruction if possible.

Immediate laryngostomy or tracheostomy (see page 160) may be necessary to save life. The exact cause of the obstruction can be sought and treated later.

Foreign Bodies in the Larynx

If the obstruction is a foreign body that can be seen, it can sometimes be hooked out with a finger, or removed by forceps. A small child can be picked up by the ankles and thumped on the back.

A large object impacted in the larynx is likely to cause acute obstruction, necessitating immediate tracheotomy. This operation may also be required to relieve the dyspnœa caused by small foreign bodies. Pins, nails and other sharp objects cause sudden pain, cough, loss of voice, and in some cases, spasm of the vocal cords to such a degree that tracheostomy is essential to enable respiration until the foreign body is removed. The spasm usually passes off if the body becomes impacted, but its movements excite fresh attacks and, sometimes, hæmoptysis. If the object is not soon removed, inflammatory œdema and abscess may follow, though several years may pass without the development of serious symptoms.

Examination by indirect (with a mirror) or direct laryngoscopy will usually establish the diagnosis. In some cases, X-rays may be required. Removal is achieved by straight forceps passed down the tube of a direct laryngoscope.

Benign Tumours of the Larynx

Innocent new growths of the larynx are comparatively common. Those that occur are papilloma, fibroma and, more rarely, lipoma and angioma.

Papilloma.—The growths are usually multiple in

DISEASES OF THE LARYNX

children. They are warty, usually pedunculated and may be white, pink or red. They appear to rest on the cords, but may grow from below and on the trachea.

Symptoms.—The symptoms are hoarseness only, unless the papillomata are multiple or very large, and then dyspnœa and stridor may occur.

Rapid recurrence often needs tracheostomy.

Fibroma is usually situated on the upper surface of the vocal cord. These growths always occur singly.

Angioma presents itself on the cords or the mucous membrane near them. It occasionally gives rise to hæmoptysis.

Treatment.—This consists of removal with laryngeal forceps passed under direct vision through a laryngoscope. The tumours are usually small and easily nipped off but an angioma may need the application of a cautery to check hæmorrhage and this should be followed by laryngofissure—the surgical splitting of the thyroid cartilage—in order to remove the growth.

Malignant Tumours of the Larynx

These are relatively uncommon but occur ten times more often in men than in women. This may be due to better oral hygiene and less abuse of the voice by women. They usually affect the middle-aged or elderly, and are of the squamous-celled carcinoma type. Metastatic deposits in the larynx are rare, and laryngeal growths themselves seldom metastasize. The growths are classified as:

1. *Intrinsic tumours*—inside the larynx. These generally arise from the vocal cords and grow slowly.

2. *Extrinsic tumours.*—These mostly commence outside the larynx and therefore are more accurately classified as pharyngeal tumours. They may develop

on the epiglottis, the aryepiglottic folds or the piriform fossa. (See page 138). Their growth is more rapid and involves the lymphatics early. They are therefore more difficult to treat and much more serious than intrinsic tumours.

Intrinsic Tumours

Symptoms.—At first, hoarseness is the only symptom. Later, when the growth spreads to the opposite cord, there is pain, cough and dyspnœa. Still later, the voice becomes a whisper, and the growth becomes extrinsic.

Extrinsic Malignant Tumours

Symptoms.—Discomfort and, later, pain on swallowing, sore throat, painful ear. Symptoms are often vague and intermittent. A node may present itself first. The voice is affected only if the growth spreads to the glottis. It causes increasing difficulty and pain on swallowing. A patient with an extrinsic malignant tumour of the larynx exhibits marked signs of cachexia.

To make a correct diagnosis of laryngeal tumour, it is frequently necessary to remove a section for examination by microscope.

Treatment of Intrinsic and Extrinsic Laryngeal Tumours

(*a*) *Intrinsic Tumours*

Early growths limited to one cord are treated by either distant radiation or implantation of radium needles. Advanced growths usually require a total laryngectomy. If glands are present, these are removed at the same time.

(*b*) *Extrinsic tumours*

The treatment of these growths is mentioned on page 125. Where complicated operations are carried out, the nursing contribution is extremely important.

DISEASES OF THE LARYNX

Sometimes no curative treatment is possible, owing to the advanced stage of the disease or the age and weakness of the patient, and sometimes the treatment attempted is unsuccessful. Even so, good nursing can help to cheer the patient considerably and reduce his discomfort.

Complications and their Treatment.—The complications which eventually terminate life are dysphagia, asphyxia, hæmorrhage or sepsis. For the increasing dysphagia, gastrostomy is sometimes performed. Should there be sudden dyspnœa and respiratory obstruction a low tracheostomy may be required, but as a rule, the obstruction comes on so gradually that the patient, who is usually in bed, is not distressed by it.

The teeth and mouth must be kept as clean as possible. Once the tumour begins to ulcerate, the mouth becomes very septic, the breath has a sickly odour, abscesses occur, and the cervical glands are enlarged and tender. Septic absorption causes rapid wasting and loss of strength. Alkaline cleansing lotions are used for the mouth, and frequent washes or sprays with a deodorant such as Sanitas. Antiseptic and deodorant throat lozenges are also helpful and are best sucked after meals.

Small amounts of liquid paraffin may be given two or three times a day, as straining from constipation must be avoided. Dulcolax suppositories are useful if constipation does occur.

In the later stages of the growth, neuralgic pain is marked. Aspirin mixtures may relieve this at first, but morphine becomes necessary in increasing doses and helps to relieve distress from other causes.

16

Operations on the larynx and pharynx

Tracheostomy

The term "tracheotomy" strictly means an opening into the trachea. "Tracheostomy" is the correct term for an opening which is to be kept patent.

The operation, by making an opening through the neck into the trachea, provides an airway in cases of impending asphyxia due to laryngeal obstruction. More recently the operation has been performed

FIG. 34.—CUFFED RADCLIFFE TRACHEOSTOMY TUBE.

increasingly for other kinds of respiratory difficulty—e.g. in paralysis, head injuries, tetanus, chronic bronchitis, bronchopneumonia, etc. The object is not only to provide assisted respiration by intermittent positive pressure, but in order to be able to aspirate secretions and prevent aspiration into the lungs. In these cases, a cuffed tracheostomy tube is used (see Fig. 34). This is made of disposable polythene. The operation may be one of two types: planned and emergency.

Planned Tracheostomy

In the great majority of cases, tracheostomy is performed under local anæsthesia, as any patient requiring the operation will be liable to respiratory difficulty with a general anæsthetic unless he can be intubated. The patient should be reassured, told that the operation will only take a few minutes, that he will feel no pain and very little discomfort. The skin of the neck, from the tip of the chin to half-way down the sternum should be shaved, washed, and prepared according to the customary requirements of the surgeon.

The instruments for tracheostomy are:

1. Tracheostomy tubes. There is widespread use of disposable tubes with wide bore and no inner tube, but non-disposable ones are still used, e.g. Durham's (see page 251), consisting of:
   - (*a*) Outer tube.
   - (*b*) Inner tube.
   - (*c*) Pilot.
   - (*d*) Tapes looped to the fittings on the outer tube, one end short and one long enough to come round the neck and tie at one side. The tube or cannula must be long enough to reach into the lumen of the trachea from the skin surface. The flanges are adjustable on the outer end of the tubes for this purpose. As long a tube as possible is used. The usual sizes are: Number 5 for an adult, 4 for an adolescent, 2 or 3 for children and 1 for infants.
2. Scalpels or small Bard-Parker's knife with blades.
3. Two small blunt hook retractors.
4. A sharp hook.
5. Tracheal dilators, e.g. Bowlby's.
6. Six pairs small artery forceps.

7. Pointed dissecting scissors.
8. Small, full-curved suture needles.
9. Full-curved skin needles.
10. Needle holder.
11. Suture material.
12. Ligatures, e.g. steel, silk, nylon.
13. Hypodermic syringe for the local anæsthetic, with reinforced bent needles.
14. Gauze swabs with X-ray opaque marker.
15. Disposable catheters for aspiration through the tracheal tube.
16. Suction apparatus, preferably electric.

Cylinders of oxygen should be at hand, and also the bronchoscopic outfit in case of necessity.

The patient lies on his back and the shoulders may be slightly raised on pillows on the operating table. A child should be pinned in a blanket. A sand-bag is placed under the shoulders so as to extend the head which must be held exactly in the midline by an assistant.

The skin having been prepared, the local anæsthetic is injected into the tissues from the level of the hyoid bone to the suprasternal notch. An incision is then made through the skin and superficial fascia transversely over the thyroid isthmus. Any bleeding vessels are clamped and the incision is then deepened to the cricoid cartilage and the tracheal rings. The isthmus of the thyroid gland may be retracted out of the way, or it may be clamped, divided and ligatured, which is the usual preference. The wound is then thoroughly dried by mopping with gauze swabs, the trachea is fixed with the sharp hook or tenaculum forceps and is incised in the midline through the third, fourth and fifth rings. Great care is taken not to cut the membranous wall at the back of the trachea. As soon as the trachea is opened, there is a hiss of air and sometimes a little spluttering, but the edges of the wound usually close

OPERATIONS ON THE LARYNX AND PHARYNX

quickly. The tracheal dilators are therefore immediately inserted. A clot of mucus is coughed out at this point, and if dyspnœa has been at all severe, the patient gives a deep sigh of relief. Frequently, an exhausted child has fallen asleep on the operating table.

The surgeon usually then trims the edges of the incision to make an oval opening through which the cannula is inserted. If the cannula is of the proper length, the shield will stand out a little from the level of the skin. The pilot is removed and the tapes are tied lightly round the neck. The wound is closed with interrupted sutures, not too close to the tube. The nurse can then release the patient's head. A dressing is applied, of about six layers of folded gauze, cut halfway down, so as to fit round the tube under the shields.

After-Care

The patient is returned to bed, and placed in a semi-recumbent or a sitting position unless this is contra-indicated by his general condition. A special nurse should be in constant attendance, night and day for a number of days depending upon the reason for operation. Beside the bed should be kept a tray or pack containing the following sterile apparatus:

An exact duplicate of the tracheostomy tube, complete with tapes.

1 pair of tracheal dilators.

1 pair of pointed scissors.

2 pairs of fine artery forceps.

1 probe.

A bowl of gauze swabs.

Fine disposable catheters, size 12.

A paper bag for used catheters.

Oxygen and suction apparatus should be available.

The room should be well ventilated, and if the air is very dry, a steam tent is beneficial.

The special duty of the nurse is to see that the airway is kept clear. Any secretion that is coughed out through the tube should be quickly but gently wiped away so that it is not sucked back into the trachea. Suction should be applied whenever there is secretion to be aspirated, using a catheter which is passed down the tracheostomy tube for 25 to 50 mm. Rattling or bubbling noises in the patient's respiration show that secretions are blocking the tube. When non-disposable tubes are used at least every hour for the first few days the nurse should remove the inner tube, and replace it with another sterilized tube. To remove it, she should steady the outer tube by pressing it against the neck with her fingers.

The outer tube is changed only by the surgeon, his assistant or the ward sister. This is done within 36 hours of the operation to remove blood clots and secretions. Afterwards, changing every 2 or 3 days is sufficient. The nurse should change the dressings as often as they become soiled. Should the outer tube become dislodged no time should be lost in replacing it with the duplicate tube which is kept in readiness. In the meantime the nurse should maintain the airway by inserting the tracheal dilators. The dilators with the blades closed are inserted from the side, the handles are then brought round to the midline and gently opened.

As there is no post-anæsthetic vomiting to be feared, the patient is able and should be encouraged to begin swallowing liquids at any time. Fluids should be given liberally and there is seldom any need for a feeding tube. Any leakage of fluid through the tube should of course be reported at once.

The nurse must realize that the patient is voiceless—he cannot call for help; a baby cannot cry aloud. Pre-printed, illustrated communication cards indicating the patient's needs are especially useful for children. A firm writing pad and pencil may be provided and later, when it is considered safe for the patient to be left without a nurse constantly at his side, he should be given a bell with a distinctive tone. The patient may be anxious and distressed at his inability to speak aloud. He should be reassured that this is only because air leaks through the tube, and that he will be able to talk well after some days by putting his finger over the opening of the tube.

Rest is important, and the patient should be disturbed as little as possible. On the other hand, he should move about early and may usually sit out of bed on the third or fourth day. The skin sutures are removed on the sixth day. After this, the sterile dressings around the tube are unnecessary. The patient is encouraged to breathe deeply and to cough, being supplied with gauze swabs or paper handkerchiefs to catch mucus. The majority of patients requiring a permanent tracheostomy are fitted with a plastic tracheostomy tube and are taught to manage this themselves. They are then able to go home, instructions being given concerning attendance at the Out-Patients' Department.

Emergency Tracheostomy

No one should be allowed to suffocate from absolute laryngeal obstruction for want of a bold attempt at tracheostomy on the part of an onlooker. It may be possible to use the instruments of an already-sterilized tracheostomy set, but if these are not accessible, the operation can be performed with a knife and a dilator (possibly improvised).

The position of the patient and the operation follow the same general lines as for a planned tracheostomy, except that there is no time for the usual skin preparation though there may be time to cleanse quickly with ether, methylated or surgical spirit, and a local anæsthetic is not necessary as the patient is unconscious or nearly so. The fingers of the operator's left hand are used to fix and identify the trachea, and no attempt is made to pick up bleeding points.

The head must be held straight since the incision must be in the midline. The trachea is identified by its ridged structure with the left index finger and is fixed in the midline with the left thumb and middle finger. When the incision has been made, a dilator must be inserted—using artery forceps or the knife handle if necessary—and the incision kept open until a tracheostomy tube can be put in. It may be necessary to apply artificial respiration and give oxygen to re-establish breathing. The severed blood vessels quickly stop bleeding with the fall of the raised pressure due to the asphyxia.

In some cases of asphyxia it may be possible and advisable to insert a bronchoscope, establish regular respiration through it and then perform an orderly tracheostomy. The operation is quite simple if the bronchoscope is in position.

Complications following Tracheostomy

1. **Surgical Emphysema.**—If the incision is made too big and air escapes round the tube, surgical emphysema may occur.

If, during the early dressings, the tracheostomy tube is incorrectly replaced, a false passage may be made which will not only cause dyspnœa but will allow air to penetrate the cervical tissues and leak downwards into the mediastinum or upwards to the head. The emphysema produces swelling and a distinctive crackling sound on palpation. Little treatment is required once the tube's position has been corrected. The air is gradually reabsorbed and the discomfort it caused soon passes. As the swelling subsides, the tapes will become loose and should be re-tied when necessary.

2. **Atelectasis** (see page 135).—This complication is

often wrongly diagnosed as pneumonia. It is completely relieved by the aspiration of the obstructive plug of mucus, blood clot or tissue by means of a sucker, through a bronchoscope.

3. **Stenosis of the Larynx or Trachea.**—Stenosis, if not the cause for which tracheostomy was performed, is most often consequent upon too high a tracheostomy. It may also be due to a badly-fitting cannula or to sepsis.

The tracheostomy should not be above the second ring of the trachea. If a patient is obliged to wear a tracheostomy tube for a long period, it should be checked to see that it fits perfectly. A plastic tube is usually provided for a patient with a permanent opening. If a badly-fitting tube is worn, or if it is not kept clean, there will be erosion of the mucous lining of the trachea, followed by inflammation and necrosis of the cartilage. Stenosis will cause hoarseness, and dyspnœa when attempts are made to remove or occlude the tracheostomy tube. For treatment see page 166.

4. **Pneumothorax**—due to injury of the pleura leading to pulmonary collapse.

Removal of a Tracheostomy Tube

The process of encouraging the patient to do without his tracheostomy tube is one requiring patience and skill. Since breathing through the nose is not as simple as breathing through the tube, the simple removal of the latter may cause panic especially in a child. First, it is necessary to make sure that breathing through the larynx is possible. The tracheostomy tube worn must be small enough to allow air from the nose to pass round it. Then the tube is partially occluded by a cork cut lengthwise in half. Special rubber corks are used, as ordinary corks are liable to break. When the patient has been able to sleep comfortably for two or three nights with such a cork, it is changed for one that occludes three-quarters of the tube, then for one occluding seven-eighths, and finally for one completely closing the tube. The tracheostomy tube is then removed and the patient continues to breathe by the normal route. If the tube has only been worn for a few weeks, the fistula quickly closes, but if it has been worn for several months, stratified epithelium will have grown over the passage and this prevents healing. Very little air leaks out but the mucus which does is most uncomfortable for the patient, and therefore a simple paring and suturing of the wound is carried out. This leaves an almost imperceptible scar.

If the detubation process takes more than 1 or 2 weeks, it points to stenosis. The treatment is dilatation, usually achieved by the insertion of rubber or plastic core moulds which are inserted via the larynx with the aid of a special introducer and a laryngoscope.

Laryngostomy

This is a temporary opening for respiration made through the cricothyroid membrane. It is occasionally used instead of tracheostomy, being quicker and less difficult, but it is not so satisfactory. If it becomes necessary to keep a tube for some time in the airway, a tracheostomy is usually performed and the laryngostomy wound allowed to close. Laryngostomy is only suitable for adults.

Local anæsthesia is employed, if time allows. The patient lies supine with the head extended and fixed. A traverse incision 25 mm long is made over the cricothyroid membrane, which is then opened transversely with a narrow knife or sharp-pointed scissors. A flat Butlin's laryngostomy tube or a small tracheostomy tube is then inserted and secured as for tracheostomy.

Laryngectomy and Pharyngolaryngectomy

These operations are most often performed for removal of malignant tumour of the larynx—occasionally for the relief of rare forms of laryngeal stenosis. In treatment of cancer of the larynx or pharynx, the operation chosen depends upon the amount of tissue involved. Growths involving the pharynx as well as the larynx are commonly removed by a laryngectomy combined with a partial pharyngectomy.

Pre-operative Treatment

The preparation of the patient is similar to that for tracheostomy, but since laryngectomy is a much more serious operation and is not an emergency procedure a longer period is devoted to improving the patient's state of nutrition and to oral hygiene. The teeth and gums must be in a healthy state, even if this means postponing the operation for a week or two. His heart, lungs, blood and urine are examined and the blood group is determined. The patient will be distressed at the thought that he will not be able to talk after the operation, but he can be assured that the structures which form his words will not be affected and that lessons in voice production can be given. These may begin before the operation. The patient is taught to swallow air into the œsophagus and bring it up again noisily, forming the sound into words with his tongue, lips, cheeks and palate. The patient is admitted several days prior to operation. It is important for him to get to know the ward staff and for them to gain his confidence. It is helpful for him to meet the speech therapist and to know about the post-operative therapy. Meeting a patient who has had a successful laryngectomy is also helpful in enabling him to adjust. The medico-social worker may need to contact the patient's employer in cases where later redeployment may be necessary. The haemoglobin is estimated. Blood is grouped and cross-matched.

On the day before operation the patient has his usual diet. Antibiotics are commenced. If the bowels have not been open, a small enema or suppository is given. A sedative is usually needed to ensure a night's sleep. On the morning of operation the face and neck are shaved and the skin cleansed with soap and water. The premedication (e.g. pethidine or morphine and atropine) is given $1\frac{1}{2}$ to 1 hour prior to operation. Morphine is contra-indicated after operation on account of its effect in producing depression of the respiratory centre.

A tracheostomy is performed in the theatre and a blood transfusion is started.

Varieties of Operation

The more common operations for the removal of laryngeal or pharyngeal tumours are:

1. Laryngofissure, or median thyrotomy — also known as partial laryngectomy.
2. Total laryngectomy.
3. Pharyngolaryngectomy.

A local anæsthetic is sometimes considered sufficient for all these operations, but fuller anæsthesia may be preferred, such as that produced by the following: cervical block, intravenous Pentothal, or gas, oxygen and ether. If there is respiratory obstruction, a rubber nasal airway may be introduced or an intranasal catheter. Bronchoscopic instruments should be prepared.

Laryngofissure

In this operation the larynx is split down the midline after a preliminary tracheostomy. The growth is removed with parts of one or both vocal cords. The larynx is then closed, the tracheostomy being kept open for approximately 24 hours.

The nursing is similar to that of tracheostomy. For the purpose of taking nourishment, the patient should be told to lean slightly forward and take a good swallow rather than to sip. No talking above a whisper should be allowed for the first few days.

Total Laryngectomy

For advanced malignant disease of the larynx, the whole organ is removed. The severed lower part of the trachea is brought up to the skin surface and sewn into position forming a permanent orifice. A feeding tube is passed through the nose into the stomach. Sometimes, an especially wide laryngectomy tube is inserted into the tracheal orifice but quite often this is left without a tube.

Post-operative Treatment

The nursing requirements are similar to those of tracheostomy with the addition of nasal feeding. There is a firm dressing over the neck wound. There may be a pack or drain in place. If the patient is not intubated, the nurse will find it necessary to remove small crusts of dried blood from around the edges of the orifice as they form. Four to eight ml of blood-stained serous discharge are expected in the first 24 hours and rather less on the second day.

The operation of laryngectomy is not usually associated with much shock, but 600 ml of blood has usually been transfused and this is followed by dextrose and saline throughout the first 24 hours. Careful watch should be kept on the patient's colour, and the rate of the pulse and the blood pressure level are recorded at $\frac{1}{2}$ hourly intervals until they remain at a satisfactory level.

As soon as the patient's condition allows he is raised to a semi-recumbent position. If he is in pain, an aspirin mixture may be ordered, to be given through the nasal feeding tube, but morphine is avoided.

Feeding is by the stomach tube and should begin as

soon as possible. Small amounts of water are given hourly. This gradually increases until he is having about 250 ml of milk and water every 2 hours. By the second day, ordinary food passed through a liquidizer fortified by extra protein and diluted with milk can be used to give a daily intake of 3000 Calories. At the end of a week the patient should be taking water by mouth. If this is tolerated well the tube can be removed and oral feeding commenced. In the early days after operation, a chart should be kept of the patient's intake and output of fluid. Frequent mouthwashes should be given.

The laryngectomy tube, if inserted, is usually removed about the tenth day after operation. The first dressing of the actual laryngectomy wound is performed by the surgeon. This may be on the second or third day. Sutures are removed by the sixth day. An antibiotic cover is generally provided for at least a week. Should there be any crusting Streptokinase spray can be used. Calamine cream can be applied to the skin around the tracheostomy to prevent soreness. It may be necessary to postpone natural feeding for some days until the wound is well healed.

When the feeding tube is removed, the patient can commence or continue learning the technique of speech by air-swallowing.

The patient is encouraged to get up and dress as soon as possible. If he can wear a collar and tie this is good for his morale. He is generally ready to go home at the end of a fortnight, and attends the Out-Patient's Department at weekly intervals for observation of his well-being and for speech therapy. He should be able to return to work after about a month. Radiotherapy may be required both pre- and post-operatively.

Pharyngolaryngectomy

This may be undertaken as a one-stage operation or a two-stage procedure. After a tracheostomy and a laryngectomy, the growth is removed from the pharynx. Skin flaps taken from the thigh as a donor area, are sutured to the edges of the cut pharynx and used to form a channel into the œsophagus. A feeding tube is passed along this channel into the stomach.

Post-operative Treatment

The nursing after pharyngolaryngectomy follows the same lines as after laryngectomy (see page 171). A great deal of saliva at first leaks from the pharyngostomy and therefore dressings need frequent changing. It is most important to clear the œsophageal tube after each feed and to make certain that it is patent before the next feed is given as the tube cannot be moved during the healing of the graft. After a few days it is usually found that fluid given by mouth will trickle down the pharyngeal gutter and leakage becomes steadily less. The feeding tube can be removed after a week and repositioned in the œsophagus behind the tracheostome. Closure should take place in 3 weeks; nasal feeding frequently follows for some days after its removal. Oral feeding can be commenced when the graft has taken and healed satisfactorily. Swallowing must be tested first. The tracheostomy is kept open for 3 or 4 days after operation. The thigh wound is treated as for a skin graft and is dressed according to the instructions of the surgeon.

Antibiotics and sulphonamides are of inestimable value in minimizing local sepsis. The patient may be ordered Vitamin C and iron tablets may be crushed and given with feeds.

Secondary closure of the pharyngostomy can be carried out after about 3 weeks, with plastic reconstruction of the swallowing tube.

17

The inhalation or ingestion of foreign bodies—endoscopy

Of all the emergencies dealt with in an Ear, Nose and Throat Department, those of the most common occurrence, apart from acute ear conditions, are due to the lodging of a foreign body in the deeper air or food passages. An appalling mortality rate existed until the beginning of this century, since when the development of special methods of diagnosis and treatment has considerably decreased it. These methods are known as *endoscopy*, the use of illuminating instruments which are introduced into the air or food passages in order to show the foreign body and facilitate its removal. The direct, or illuminated laryngoscope has already been referred to. Through it, other instruments such as a bronchoscope or forceps can be passed. An œsophagoscope is used to illuminate and remove objects in the œsophagus.

Generally speaking, foreign bodies impacted in the trachea, bronchi and œsophagus, if not removed, ultimately prove fatal from such causes as lung abscess or mediastinal infection. In almost every case the offending object can be removed through the mouth by endoscopy. Waiting for spontaneous expulsion is dangerous; blind methods of removal are extremely dangerous.

Foreign Body in the Larynx

This has been discussed in a previous chapter (page 156).

Foreign Body in the Trachea

In tracheal obstruction, the spasm of the larynx is much less than that occurring in laryngeal obstruction, but the stridor caused by the dyspnœa accompanies both inspiration and expiration. Should the obstruction be due to an inhaled foreign body, the choking attack which occurs as the object passes through the larynx ceases as it falls into the trachea, but a harsh cough persists and the breathing is laborious. The patient sits forward with the head flexed in an attempt to ease the strain on the trachea. If the foreign body is movable, the cough is paroxysmal. The diagnosis may be confirmed by X-rays or by endoscopy. A longer tube is required than for laryngoscopy. Removal may be made by tracheostomy, should endoscopy not be available.

Foreign Body in the Bronchus

An inhaled object is a common cause of bronchial obstruction. As foreign bodies may be of all shapes, sizes and consistency, the conditions to which they give rise when lodged in a bronchus vary a great deal. The size of the foreign body in relation to the age of the patient is important, as upon this depends the site of impaction and consequently the area of lung that may be affected. Peas and beans, which have frequently been inhaled by children, swell rapidly, causing acute inflammation and œdema of the mucosa, with consequent dyspnœa. Should there be obstruction of a main bronchus, complete collapse (atelectasis) of that lung may follow. Alternatively, the object may set up a ball-valve action, allowing air to pass it on inspiration, but not on expiration. Emphysema—the presence of air outside the air passages—then occurs. The patient has an asthmatic wheeze and feeling of tightness in the chest. An unsuspected foreign body—perhaps the patient had a choking fit during the inhalation of the object which was then drawn into a smaller bronchus—may give rise to bronchiectasis or lung abscess. Foreign bodies are more likely to be inhaled into the right bronchus than into the left, as the right is more nearly a continuation of the trachea than is the left. It is also slightly larger than the left bronchus.

Once the foreign body has been removed, and bronchoscopic aspiration carried out, it is remarkable how quickly the patient gets well.

Swallowed Foreign Bodies

Patients frequently come or are brought into hospital with clear histories of having swallowed objects of various shapes and sizes. The œsophagus has a surprising capacity of distension and cases have been reported in which a complete dental plate has been swallowed during sleep.

Sometimes quite small objects become arrested, and sharp ones can cause much damage. For example, open safety pins with points uppermost, sharp irregular bones or brooches may pierce the œsophageal wall or cause a tear unless they are removed with great care. The great majority of foreign bodies are arrested at the uppermost constriction. In this situation, coins stick transversely.

Foreign Body in the Œsophagus

Symptoms.—There is usually a feeling of something sticking. Should the object be sharp, for example a sharp bone, there is actual pain on swallowing. Occasionally, there is dyspnœa, wheezing or cough due to compression of the air passages from behind or from trickling of secretion into the larynx.

Treatment.—An X-ray examination should be carried out before attempting to remove a foreign body, and a barium swallow is sometimes given if a non-opaque object is suspected. When the site of impaction has been ascertained, œsophagoscopy should be undertaken. The nurse should prepare a complete set of bronchoscopic as well as œsophageal tubes and instruments, in case of need. The foreign body having been located through the œsophagoscope, it is carefully extracted with suitable forceps.

Endoscopy

Endoscopy is carried out in an operating theatre. There is frequently one attached to the Out-Patient Department of the Ear, Nose and Throat Unit for such purpose.

The preparation of the patient is similar for all endoscopy of the respiratory and alimentary tracts.

Unless the case is one of extreme urgency, the usual pharyngeal and laryngeal examinations are made, the lungs are tested by auscultation for air entry and the œsophagus for swallowing function.

The patient is given a general or a local anæsthetic according to the size of the instrument used. For both types of anæsthesia, the stomach should be empty to avoid vomiting. If general anæsthesia is desired, a basal anæsthetic followed by gas and oxygen is most satisfactory. Before local anæsthesia, which is frequently preferred, especially for bronchoscopy as then the patient is able to co-operate with the surgeon, the patient is usually given an injection, such as morphine 16 mg, scopolamine 0.5 mg and atropine 0.6 mg. About 1 ml of 10 per cent. solution of cocaine hydrochloride is then sprayed on the fauces and pharynx. A laryngeal applicator is tipped with wool moistened in the cocaine solution and applied to the inner surface of both lips, over the base of the tongue, over the posterior pharyngeal wall, the laryngeal aspect of the epiglottis and so into each piriform fossa where the main sensory nerve runs.

After anæsthesia has been produced, the patient may sit astride a stool and hold his chin forward and head tilted back, but the recumbent position is generally more satisfactory and comfortable. The patient lies on his back on the operating table with his shoulders as far as the middle of the scapulæ projecting over the end. An adjustable head-rest is usually fitted to the table—if not, an assistant supports the head in the same position as described for the seated patient. The head must always be kept exactly in the midline.

Direct Laryngoscopy

Various sizes of laryngoscope should be at hand. The nurse should see that a reserve of electric bulbs is available and that the electric connections are in order. Suction apparatus will be needed, as accumulated saliva will trickle down the trachea and cause coughing if not aspirated. Swallowing is almost impossible with the laryngoscope in position. Aspiration is carried out either through a channel in the laryngoscope or through an independent tube. Tracheostomy instruments should be in readiness if a foreign body is to be removed, lest it be dislodged and fall into the trachea. All instruments used in endoscopy should be sterile. Sterilization in a formalin cabinet is a satisfactory method, especially for the illuminating instruments. They can be stored in the cabinet and should be rinsed in sterile water before use.

By means of the direct laryngoscope, a brilliantly illuminated image of the larynx can be obtained. The spatula end of the instrument is passed over the tongue until the epiglottis is identified. The epiglottis is then lifted forward and the glottis and cords exposed. Beyond these can be seen the trachea, and one or both the bronchial orifices. The laryngoscope is usually passed on through the glottis to examine the sub-glottic area and the trachea. It is then slightly withdrawn and passed into the laryngopharynx to show the posterior wall of the larynx. Laryngoscopy may now be carried out through an operating microscope.

Bronchoscopy

For the introduction of a bronchoscope, a laryngoscope with a removable slide is first passed. The bronchoscope is a long slender tube which may be single or have one extension tube telescoping into the other. There are numerous perforations in the distal part of the tube to allow air to pass in and out. A watch spring is fitted to the proximal end of the extension tube. This spring is engraved with a centimetre scale to enable the surgeon to read off the total length of the tube which has been introduced.

The surgeon passes the laryngoscope and holds it with his left hand. The bronchoscope is held in his right hand and passed through the laryngoscope. When the surgeon sees the vocal cords abduct during inspiration, he slips the slanted end of the bronchoscope between the two cords with a slightly rotary motion. The slide which forms part of the barrel of the laryngoscope is pushed up and the laryngoscope removed, leaving the bronchoscope with its end free in the trachea. The tube can then be carefully moved down and rotated in order to obtain different views of the bronchial tree.

Œsophagoscopy

An œsophagoscope is similar to a sigmoidoscope, being a much larger instrument than the bronchoscope. The common type has a drainage canal in order to aspirate secretion without interruption during œsophagoscopy. An œsophageal speculum is necessary, as the lumen of the œsophagus must be located before the œsophagoscope is passed into it. Thereafter, œsophagoscopy resembles bronchoscopy. Local anæsthesia may be supplemented by intravenous Pentothal, particularly if the passage is difficult due to long upper teeth.

Gastroscopy

The stomach may be inspected through an œsophagoscope. Frequently, a flexible gastroscope is used for this purpose.

Precautions to be taken after direct peroral endoscopy are concerned with the absence of the cough reflex and are dealt with in the section on cocaine (see page 41).

18

Diseases of the œsophagus

Patients with such disorders are frequently admitted to an Ear, Nose and Throat Department as the necessary investigations include œsophagoscopy which is a technique in which the laryngologist specializes.

Œsophageal diseases, apart from impacted foreign bodies (see page 176) are classified into:

(*a*) Neuromuscular disorders — diverticulitis and achalasia.

(*b*) Strictures from fibrosis—e.g. following burns or peptic ulcers.

(*c*) Strictures from malignant tissue.

Neuromuscular Disorders of the Œsophagus

Achalasia or Cardiospasm.—In this condition, the œsophagus gradually, over many years, becomes dilated and hypertrophied and develops an obstruction at its lower end. The cause is unknown but thought to be due to inco-ordination of the autonomic nerve supply. The sufferers are usually women.

Symptoms.—A gradually increasing difficulty of swallowing leads to emaciation. There is an unpleasant odour to the breath as the dilated œsophagus contains undigested and decomposing food and liquid.

Signs.—Examination by X-rays after a barium meal has been swallowed will show the lower end of the œsophagus to be dilated, becoming sigmoid in advanced cases. Obstruction at the cardiac sphincter, where the œsophagus enters the stomach will also be shown.

If an œsophagoscope be passed after suction of the contents of the dilated œsophagus, the mucous membrane will appear inflamed and ulcerated. Malignant change in the ulcers sometimes occurs.

Treatment.—The nurse will give regular evening washouts, using a funnel and tube and normal saline. These will help to improve the condition of the mucous membrane. The cardiospasm may be relieved by repeated dilatation by means of swallowing a Hurst's bougie, which is a long rubber tube containing mercury. If operative treatment is decided upon, the patient is transferred to a ward for thoracic surgery. In Heller's operation a thoracic approach is made and the lower end of the œsophagus freed. The muscle fibres are then divided in a manner similar to Rammstedt's operation on the pyloric sphincter.

Pharyngeal Pouch.—A pressure pouch, often termed an "œsophageal diverticulum" but being truly a portion of the pharyngeal mucosa and connective tissue, becomes squeezed out between the fibres of the inferior constrictor muscles and sags down behind the œsophagus. The cause is thought to be inco-ordination between the sympathetic and parasympathetic nerve supplies.

Symptoms.—The symptoms are dysphagia, caused by the pressure on the back of the œsophagus by the food in the pouch, and regurgitation of the undigested food. The majority of patients are elderly, emaciated men. The condition and symptoms increase gradually. Often a gurgling sound can be obtained by pressure with the fingers on the swelling which appears in the neck after eating.

Diagnosis is made from the distinctive signs and symptoms and by radiography. Œsophagoscopy is usually performed in order to inspect and confirm the condition.

Treatment.—The treatment consists of washing out the pouch using a funnel and tube, and by excision of the pouch, approaching it through the side of the neck.

DISEASES OF THE ŒSOPHAGUS

After operation, tube feeding is required for about a week.

Alternatively, the "spur" between the pouch and the œsophagus can be destroyed by electro-coagulation applied through an endoscope (Dohlman's operation).

Burns of the Œsophagus

Burns from swallowing hot liquids are rare, but occasionally corrosives are swallowed by accident or intent and cause chemical burns of the œsophagus. Household ammonia, caustic soda disinfectant solution, and the sulphuric acid used in accumulators are examples of fluids that are sometimes taken in mistake for water. The corrosive effect is usually, but not always, exerted on the lips, tongue and pharynx as well as on the œsophagus. Sometimes the fluid passes quickly into the stomach and the burning of the œsophagus is very shallow, but if it lingers in the œsophagus the damage caused is very severe.

The diagnosis is usually made on the evidence of the patient or parents, and by the burns of the mouth. Weeks or months later, scarring leads to stricture formation.

Treatment.—The first-aid treatment consists of neutralizing an alkali with weak vinegar, and an acid with magnesia or sodium bicarbonate solution. The patient must be encouraged to drink whichever fluid is required, in spite of pain on swallowing. Demulcents such as milk or beaten egg are given. Sometimes a copious flow of saliva accumulates in the mouth as the patient is afraid to swallow. This may be aspirated, and then a little bismuth powder is often sprinkled on the tongue and washed down with water. This should be repeated every half-hour for a few days, less often after that. Water must be given regularly and dehydration avoided. Steroids are given early to lessen fibrosis and penicillin to limit the infection to sloughing.

After about 2 weeks, very gentle œsophagoscopy is carried out every week or 10 days in the attempt to prevent narrowing of the œsophagus by scar tissue, which, however, is a common sequel to burning.

A modern line of treatment is to expose the pharynx by incision in the neck and to create a pharyngostome. A feeding tube of large size is inserted and left in place for perhaps 2 to 3 months. Antibiotics and cortisone are given to limit sepsis and scarring.

Non-malignant Stenosis of the Œsophagus

This is commonly due to swallowing corrosive fluids, but may follow ulceration caused by syphilis or other disease. The stricture is most apt to form at the narrowing caused by the crossing of the left bronchus but there are frequently other strictures present wherever ulcers heal.

Symptom.—The symptom is regurgitation of food.

Treatment.—If the stricture is severe, gastrostomy is necessary, after which, the stricture may be excised and the œsophageal stump anastomosed with the stomach. This operation will be carried out in a department for general or thoracic surgery.

If the stricture is patent, the treatment consists of gradual and repeated dilatation. This is frequently done by passing bougies through an œsophagoscope. Another method is to give the patient a silk thread to swallow. Gastrostomy is performed and the end of the thread is brought out through the incision. On the silk are threaded three graduated metal olives and an endless chain is made. The olives are swallowed, brought out of the gastrostomy, cleaned and reswallowed. The treatments are repeated at intervals of a few days, the olives gradually being increased in size. Quite small children can be induced to swallow the olives especially if they are smeared with something sweet.

Peptic Ulceration of the Œsophagus

A peptic ulcer in the œsophagus occurs at its lower end from an upward escape of gastric juice from the stomach. This is common in patients who have a diaphragmatic hernia of the stomach due to a congenital shortening of the œsophagus or to increased abdominal pressure, together with a degeneration of the fibres encircling the œsophagogastric junction.

Symptoms.—The symptoms are dysphagia in addition to those of a gastric ulcer. They are intermittent but progressive. The dysphagia is for solid food. The pain is in the epigastrium and usually penetrates through to the back and often to the left shoulder. Attacks come on shortly after meals or in assuming a recumbent position. Vomiting may bring relief; so will the taking of alkali. Patients usually choose to sleep in the sitting position. Long-continued ulceration will result in narrowing of the œsophagus by scar tissue.

The diagnosis is made by an X-ray study after swallowing barium. Œsophagoscopy is important to show the amount of ulceration and stenosis present, and to exclude carcinoma.

Treatment.—The medical treatment is largely dietetic. Stricture is treated by dilatation through an œsophagoscope, or more often, since the disease is progressive, by operation.

Carcinoma of the Œsophagus

Cancer of the œsophagus is a comparatively common form of malignant disease although it seems now to be rarer than it was formerly. It is a most distressing condition, but of recent years surgery of the œsophagus has made great advances, and if the carcinoma can be diagnosed reasonably early, a radical resection of the affected area can be achieved, and in addition, restoration of the alimentary tract is established by means of an œsophagogastric or œsophagojejunal anastomosis or by the use of artificial grafts.

Symptoms.—The typical patient is an elderly or middle-aged man, very thin but of good colour, who for some months has suffered from increasing dysphagia. He complains that the food sticks at some point according to the site of the obstruction. The food is often regurgitated after a few minutes. It is undigested, not acid to litmus and has not reached the stomach. The dysphagia is intermittent in carcinoma of the œsophagus and is often ignored by the patient until the taking of solid food is impossible. Pain is usually a late symptom of the disease, so that the malignant condition is rarely discovered early. Therefore, any reported abnormality of swallowing should be investigated by X-rays, the œsophagoscope, and if a lesion is seen, by biopsy and examination of the specimen.

Treatment is carried out in a ward for general surgery and will not be described in detail here. Gastrostomy is best avoided, and if a radical resection is not advisable, radiotherapy can give some temporary relief. Sometimes Souttar's tube, or similar device made from plastic material, is inserted to enable the patient whose case is hopeless to swallow with relative comfort.

Section V: The Ear

19

Anatomy of the ear

The ear is anatomically divided into three parts:

The Outer Ear, consisting of the auricle or pinna and the external auditory meatus, which is a passage leading to the ear drum;

The Middle Ear, which is a roughly spherical cavity about the size of a large pea, situated within the temporal bone, internal to the ear drum;

The Inner Ear, which is situated deeply within the temporal bone. It is connected via the internal auditory meatus with the central nervous system by the auditory (8th cranial) nerve, which has two distinct parts, the cochlear concerned with hearing and the vestibular concerned with the sense of balance.

The External Ear

The Auricle, except in the lobe, is made up of an irregular plate of elastic cartilage covered by skin. It is attached to the temporal bone by ligaments and is continuous with the cartilage of the auditory meatus. There are some muscular attachments, but very little movement of the external ear occurs in man; it is purely ornamental. In other animals, such as the dog, the auricle is moved in order to catch sound waves. On the anterior surface of the auricle, the skin adheres closely to the cartilage, which accounts for the frequent occurrence of hæmatoma following injury of this surface, but on the posterior surface it is looser.

The auricle is supplied with blood from the posterior auricular artery behind, and the superficial temporal

188 EAR, NOSE AND THROAT NURSING

artery in front. The superficial position of the vessels in the thin skin and the lack of subcutaneous tissue and fat, make the auricle particularly susceptible to frostbite.

Fig. 35.—The Auricle of the Ear.

The sensory nerves supplying the auricle are branches from the mandibular division of the trigeminal nerve, the lesser occipital and great auricular nerves from the cervical plexus, and the auricular branch of the vagus nerve. The muscles of the auricle are supplied by the facial nerve.

Different parts of the auricle are described by special names which are shown in Fig. 35. The free lobe of the ear is characteristic of man.

The External Auditory Meatus begins as a funnel-shaped opening in the auricle and leads inwards to the temporal bone, where it is closed by the tympanic (or drum-like) membrane. The latter is placed obliquely so that the canal of an adult is about 26 mm long on the superoposterior wall and 32 mm long on the antero-inferior wall. Wax frequently collects in the lower corner so formed. The meatus is in the shape of an elongated and twisted S, the direction being first upward, inward and forward. It soon bends backward and inward, then downward inward and backward. To straighten and make the drum visible, it is necessary

ANATOMY OF THE EAR

to pull the auricle upward and backward. The outer third, or rather more, of the auditory canal is cartilaginous, the remainder lies in the temporal bone. The entire canal is lined by skin. There are two constrictions in the canal, one near the medial end of the cartilaginous portion, and one in the osseous portion.

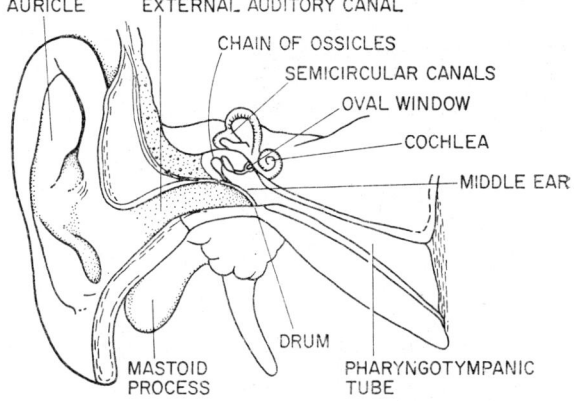

FIG. 36.—VIEW OF THE RIGHT EAR WITH THE EXTERNAL AND MIDDLE EAR SEEN IN SECTION DURING SWALLOWING.
(Except when swallowing, the mouth of the pharyngotympanic tube is closed.)

Near the auricle, the skin lining the canal is set with hairs, while within, in the subcutaneous tissue of the cartilaginous portion are numerous ceruminous glands which secrete wax. The hairs help to prevent the entrance of insects, and by means of the wax insects and bacteria are entangled. Absence of wax occurs in disease. An accumulation of wax may block the passage and cause deafness. In the bony portion of the external auditory meatus the skin is thin, devoid of hairs and contains very few wax glands. The shortness of the meatus in children, before the skull bones have fully ossified, must be remembered when examining with an aural speculum, lest the ear drum be damaged.

The Middle Ear

The middle ear or tympanic cavity is an air-containing cavity, hollowed out in the substance of the temporal

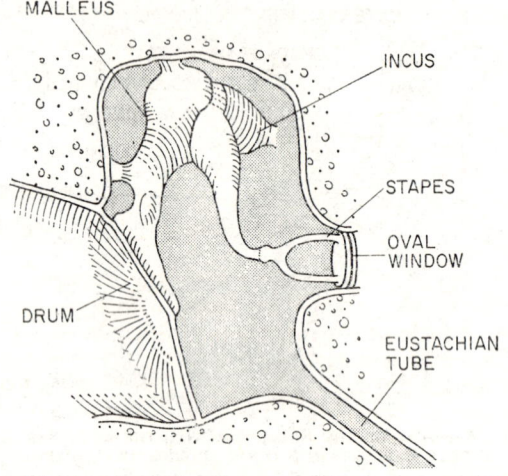

Fig. 37.—The Right Ear Drum, the Malleus and the Incus (Internal View).

bone and is separated from the outer ear by the tympanic membrane or ear drum.

The Tympanic Membrane.—This is an exceedingly thin, pearly grey, semi-transparent membrane, almost circular, having a vertical diameter of about 10 mm and a horizontal diameter of 7.5 mm. Its circumference is slightly thickened and forms a fibrocartilaginous ring by which it is attached to the medial end of the external auditory meatus. The inner surface of the membrane is convex, and to the point of greatest convexity is attached the tip of the malleus, the first of the chain of ossicles which crosses the middle ear. Below this point, on examining the ear from the meatus by reflected light, a brightly illuminated "cone of light" can be seen over the antero-inferior quadrant of the membrane. Here the drum presents a plane surface to the light rays, with no structure to obscure its translucency. There is a small, somewhat triangular area in the upper part of the ear drum which is loose (called Shrapnell's membrane) but the main part of the drum is tightly stretched. Although the drum is so thin, it consists of 4 layers:

1. The outer layer of stratified epithelium, derived from the skin lining the external auditory meatus;
2. A layer of radiating white connective tissue fibres;
3. A layer of circular fibres, thicker around the circumference;
4. The mucous membrane lining the middle ear.

In the flaccid part of the drum, the fibrous tissue is absent, and therefore this is the weakest part.

The roof of the middle ear is formed by a thin plate of bone—part of the anterior surface of the petrous portion of the temporal bone—which separates it from the cranial cavity. On the *inner wall*, there are two small openings, the oval window (fenestra ovalis) and the round window (fenestra rotunda). Both of these are closed by membranes. They lead to the internal ear— the oval window to the vestibule and the round window to the cochlea.

From the anterior wall, near the floor of the middle ear, passing forwards and inwards, is the pharyngo-tympanic tube, long known as the *Eustachian tube*. This tube is about 40 mm long and leads into the nasopharynx. Through it, air enters the middle ear. The posterior third of the tube is surrounded by the temporal bone, and the anterior two-thirds are partly cartilaginous and partly fibrous. The tube is closed except in the action of swallowing. Then, the flaccid walls of the tube are pulled apart by the action of one of the swallowing muscles. A cold in the nose sometimes spreads up the pharyngotympanic tube and the swollen mucous membrane blocks the tube. As a result the air in the middle ear cannot be renewed; it becomes absorbed by the blood in the capillaries, and the pressure of the air outside the tympanic membrane is no longer counterbalanced by the air within. The membrane is then pulled in tightly and cannot vibrate. This causes the deafness that is so common in people with heavy colds. In children the pharyngotympanic tube is more horizontal than in adults and therefore infection can pass from the nose to the middle ear more easily.

Mastoid Air Cells.—The middle ear cavity also opens into an air space in the mastoid process, known as the mastoid antrum, which in turn opens into other air cells. These air spaces develop in growing bone in the same way as the paranasal sinuses and are similarly lined with mucous membrane. The mastoid process is recognizable as a bony prominence towards the end of the second year. In an adult, whose mastoid air cells are completely developed, the prominence is large and rounded. Frequently, however, the development is retarded, the air cells small or absent, and the process small. The bony roof of the mastoid antrum is extremely thin, especially in a child, and infection in the middle ear and mastoid antrum may spread to the dura mater of the cranial fossa.

Auditory Ossicles.—Across the cavity of the middle ear are strung three exquisitely small bones called the auditory ossicles. These are: the malleus or hammer, the incus or anvil, and the stapes or stirrup, being named after objects they resemble. They are attached to each other by ligaments. The rounded head of the malleus is jointed to a hollow in the incus, and the long

ANATOMY OF THE EAR

arm of the incus is similarly jointed to the stapes. The long handle of the hammer bone is attached to the ear drum, and the plate of the stirrup is fixed to the membrane which closes the oval window. The line of attachment of the malleus is visible on the eardrum when examined through the external meatus. All three ossicles are covered by thin mucous membrane continuous with that lining the walls of the middle ear. There is a recess in the middle ear, lying above and behind the head of the malleus and the body of the incus, called the *attic* or *epitympanic recess*. This leads

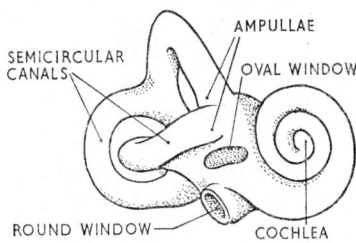

FIG. 38.—THE BONY LABYRINTH.

into the mastoid antrum and is important in cases of infection of the middle ear.

Sound waves, causing the ear drum to vibrate, are generally thought to be amplified by the chain of ossicles and transmitted to the oval window. From here, they travel through the inner ear and return to the round window. The physiology of hearing will be further described in the next chapter.

The Internal Ear

The internal ear, or labyrinth, comprises a series of cavities and canals in the petrous portion of the temporal bone. The bony canals and spaces are called the *bony labyrinth*. They are lined with periosteum and enclose the *membranous labyrinth*. The bony labyrinth is formed of three layers; an outer periosteal layer, a middle layer derived from the cartilage surrounding the embryonic membranous labyrinth, and an inner layer of endosteum. The inner layer has no blood vessels and is of ivory-like hardness. The adjacent side of the middle layer is also dense, but the external layer next to the periosteum is of looser texture. In the disease called otosclerosis, the changes in bone occur in this layer.

The different parts of the bony labyrinth are: the vestibule, the three semicircular canals, and the cochlea.

Fig. 39.—Section of the Right Osseous Cochlea and Internal Auditory Meatus.

The Vestibule lies medially to the tympanic cavity, its lateral wall being perforated by the oval and round windows. It is a small irregular cavity, and the cochlea leads into it from the front and the semicircular canals from behind.

The Semicircular Canals are very small hoops of bone, each forming about two-thirds of a circle, and having a diameter of one millimetre except at one end where it dilates into an "ampulla". The canals are set at right angles to each other, in different planes. Their non-ampullated ends join to make a common entrance in the medial wall of the vestibule. The ampullæ of the superior and lateral canals have their openings into the vestibule above the oval windows, whilst the posterior ampulla opens into it below the oval window.

The Bony Cochlea is a flattened cone, about 1 cm at its base. It is formed of a central column, the modiolus, around which a hollow spiral tube makes two and a half turns, like a snail shell. A delicate spiral shelf of bone projects from the modiolus into the canal and winds upwards to the apex. The shelf reaches about half-way across the canal, and partially divides it into two. The division is completed by a membrane called

Fig. 40.—The Membranous Labyrinth (Diagrammatic).

the basilar membrane, and the two canals communicate at the apex of the cochlea. In the modiolus are small openings through which pass branches of the cochlear nerve. The base of the cochlea has three openings: the opening into the vestibule, the round window, and a minute duct through which connection is made with the subarachnoid space.

The Membranous Labyrinth.—This structure lies within the bony labyrinth, but is very much smaller. The space between it and the surrounding bone is occupied by *perilymph*, which is a fluid identical in composition, and confluent with, the cerebrospinal fluid. The membranous labyrinth contains fluid called *endolymph*, and in its walls the filaments of the auditory nerve are distributed. Inside the semicircular canals the membranous labyrinth closely follows the shape of the bone; in the vestibule it forms two sacs called the *utricle* and the *saccule*; in the cochlea it is arranged as a third spiral tube lying along the outer wall of the cochlea. (The double bony spiral of the cochlea contains perilymph, the membranous duct contains endolymph.)

FIG. 41.—A PAIR OF RODS OF CORTI.

The various parts of the membranous labyrinth form a closed system of channels which communicate with each other. In the case of the utricle, saccule and semi-circular canals, the inner surface of the membranous labyrinth shows patches of neuro-epithelial tissue—one in the utricle, one in the saccule and one in each ampulla. These patches consist of supporting cells and sensory cells with hair-like processes which project into the endolymph. Around these hair cells terminate the branches (peripheral processes) of the vestibular nerve—the central processes of this nerve mostly end in the medulla oblongata (vestibular nuclei) and in the cerebellum. Here secondary connections are made which govern the equilibrium of the body.

Within the cochlea lies the *organ of Corti*, the receiving apparatus for hearing. It is formed of highly specialized epithelial cells, making a tunnel of tiny arched rods, resting on the basilar membrane. On either side of the tunnel are the sensory cells with hair-

ANATOMY OF THE EAR 197

like processes. It has been estimated that there are nearly 10,000 of these rods, and twice that number of hair cells, within the spiral membranous labyrinth of the cochlea. The cochlear nerve fibres which terminate round the hair cells, pass into the medulla oblongata

FIG. 42.—THE FACIAL CANAL IN THE TEMPORAL BONE.

and thence to the principal auditory centres in the cerebrum. The cochlear and the vestibular nerves join before leaving the inner ear to form the auditory (8th cranial) nerve. Although the cochlear nerve is that of hearing, and the vestibular nerve that of balance, the two have some connections, and both can influence motor cells in the spinal cord.

The Facial Nerve in Relation to the Ear

The facial nerve, in part of its course, lies in so intimate a relation to the ear, that it is often involved in diseases of and operations upon the latter.

The 7th cranial (facial) and the 8th cranial (auditory) nerves emerge side by side from the brain at the lower border of the pons, and together enter the internal auditory meatus. At the bottom of the meatus, the nerve enters the facial canal, a bony groove in the temporal bone. This groove is first directed laterally between the vestibule and the cochlea of the ear, then it passes into the aditus, downwards in the posterior wall of the middle ear and so into the mastoid process.

Finally, the facial nerve emerges through the stylomastoid foramen (see Fig. 42), and supplies the muscles of the face. It is therefore below and in front of the inner part of the mastoid antrum. Facial paralysis may result from caries of the bony wall of the middle ear.

In operative treatment, great care is necessary to avoid damaging the nerve.

In an infant, the mastoid process has not developed, so that the mastoid antrum lies above rather than behind the middle ear, and the facial nerve emerges from the stylomastoid foramen beneath the skin, unprotected by the mastoid process. An incautious incision down to the bone may then cut the nerve.

A short distance before the facial nerve leaves the bone, a branch is given off to the middle ear, to a small muscle inserted into the stapes. This muscle is caused to contract reflexly in response to very loud sounds and so is able to protect the organ of Corti from noise injury to some extent.

20
Physiology of the ear. Deafness

The functions of the ear are hearing and balance. Either or both of these are disturbed in diseases of the ear, and in order to understand them, the previous chapter should be studied. The physiology of the ear is briefly considered here.

The Physiology of Hearing

As with the other senses, hearing depends on four principal factors. There must be a stimulus, a receptor organ and a nerve pathway leading from the organ to the brain. In the temporal lobe of the brain there is an auditory area which receives the sensation of hearing and round it is an area which interprets what is heard.

In the sensory organ are the end-organs of the nerve fibres which, carrying the impulses along, form the nerves. The ear is the receptor organ of sound, and in the innermost part, the internal ear, is the organ of Corti (see Fig. 41). This is composed of little hair-like structures, the end-organs of the sensory fibres, which are supported by the basilar membrane, a continuation from the bony platform spiralling round the central modiolus of the cochlea. The fibres pass via the bony ledge and the modiolus to the base of the cochlea and emerge as the auditory part of the eighth nerve through the internal auditory meatus.

The external auditory meatus and the middle ear are constructed to carry the sound waves to the inner ear. Sound waves are disturbances in the air produced by a sounding body, e.g. a plucked violin string, a banging door or the human voice, very like the ripples raised on the surface of a pond if a stone is dropped into it. The ripples or vibrations are counted in numbers per second, the greater the number the higher the pitch, and vice versa. It is essential for the good conduction of sound that atmospheric pressure is equal on either side of the tympanic membrane separating the external from the middle ear. The air in the middle ear comes up the pharyngotympanic tube (Eustachian tube), hence a blocked pharyngotympanic tube can produce deafness.

The waves of sound striking the tympanic membrane cause it to vibrate, and this movement is transmitted across the middle ear, usually through the body of the malleus and the short arm of the incus to the stapes. The footplate of the stapes, pushing the oval window in and out, sets up a travelling wave in the perilymph and along the basilar membrane. The perilymph is separated from the endolymph only by the upper membrane of the scala media, the membrane of Reissner. The swell therefore sets up a motion in the endolymph which rocks the basilar membrane and pulls on the sensitive end-organs of Corti. The wave ends at the round window which gives to accommodate it. Sound may reach the cochlea by vibrations conducted through the bones of the head, but a much greater intensity is needed for bone conduction than for air conduction.

Sensations of sound are distinguished by their loudness, their pitch and their quality. Loudness depends upon the amplitude of vibrations; pitch, as already explained, upon the number of vibrations in a given time; quality, upon the regularity of the vibrations. A noise is the result of irregular vibrations, and a musical note is produced when the vibrations are orderly. The organ of Corti is responsible for separating the mixed vibrations which fall on the ear, and converting each set into the corresponding nerve impulses.

For sound waves to pass freely through the ear, several factors are essential:

1. The tympanic membrane must be able to vibrate.
2. The pressure in the middle ear must equal that of the atmosphere.
3. The ossicles must be able to move.
4. The oval window and the round window must both be able to yield to the waves passing through the perilymph in the labyrinth of the inner ear.

Tinnitus is the sensation of hearing in the absence of external sound. It varies in pitch and character and may become extremely distressing. The cause may be anywhere in the path of transmission. It may be a lesion of the cochlea or some part of the auditory nerve and the condition may occur in many ear diseases or arise from the over-use of drugs such as quinine and the sodium salicylates including aspirin.

Noise

There is considerable variation in the way in which different people react to noise. A sound volume which is acceptable to one person can be totally unacceptable to another. The factors which influence response to noise are both numerous and varied. The extrovert type of person who likes excitement may well find that music played at full volume is not only acceptable, but also pleasurable, while someone of more introvert nature, who is quiet and more reserved, may find the same volume quite intolerable. Similarly, the same loud music which gives pleasure to a young person, may well be an annoying noise to somebody in an older age group. Susceptibility to noise can also be affected by its cause. A man repairing or altering his home may not notice the noise created by his activity, but his neighbour who is trying to rest will not agree that the sounds are of reasonable level.

The judgement of sound intensity is subjective, and consequently the effects of noise are diverse. It can produce fatigue, frustration, irritation or considerable emotional disturbance. In certain instances it can result in actual damage to the ear and hearing loss. Exposure to noise of high intensity for a short period can result in auditory fatigue, which causes temporary deafness lasting several hours. Alternatively, in rare instances, it can rupture the tympanic membrane. This type of damage usually heals rapidly or is surgically repaired. Prolonged exposure to intense noise can result in damage to the inner ear. Such exposure damages the hair cells of the organ of Corti within the cochlea. There is decreased ability to hear higher pitched tones. At first the individual is unaware of this loss, and with continued exposure, further damage occurs. There will be difficulty in hearing speech in the higher frequencies (i.e. the consonants) of normal conversation. In consequence, the person misinterprets words and is unable to understand conversation. Later in life deafness due to advancing years may well aggravate the disability. Hearing aids are of little help to a noise-deaf person because they only amplify the sound without clarifying reception. In order to communicate, it is advisable to face the affected person and speak to them slowly and clearly without raising the voice unduly.

Where a person is subjected to continuous noise precautionary measures should be taken. For example, in industry a variety of methods of noise reduction are employed on machinery, which may be enclosed or muffled with acoustic, absorbent material. Where noise is a definite occupational hazard, ear muffs or plugs are provided to give protection. Not only are the employees encouraged to wear these, but the reason for their provision is carefully explained.

The Physiology of Balance

The ear is the organ of balance as well as of hearing. The receptor organs in this case are the semicircular

PHYSIOLOGY OF THE EAR

canals, the saccule and the utricle. They are continuous with the membranous part of the cochlea and also contain endolymph.

The vestibular portion of the eighth nerve contains the nerve fibres running from the end-organs, which lie in the ampullæ of the semicircular canals, and the maculæ of the saccule and the utricle (see Fig. 40), to the cerebellum, which co-ordinates the muscle movements controlling posture and balance. Two types of sensation are involved. The maculæ are stimulated by alterations in the *position* of the head and supply some of the information necessary for regulating the muscle tone on which posture depends.

The semicircular canals are concerned with *movements* of the head. They lie horizontally, vertically and obliquely, and the endolymph filling them follows the movements of the head. Attached to the hair cells lining the membrane and projecting into this fluid are small particles of calcium carbonate called *otoliths*. The nerve endings in the ampullæ are sensitive to alterations in fluid pressure produced by circular and rotary movements. The resulting stimuli travel along the nerve fibres to the cerebellum. The cerebellar response involves the organizing of the showers of impulses passing out from the cerebral cortex to opposing groups of muscles, so that whatever their activity, balance is maintained.

Hence injury or disease involving the labyrinths of the inner ear, e.g. Ménière's disease, will affect the power of balance. The patient suffers from a sense of falling or rotation (vertigo) which he attempts to counteract by muscular movements and therefore he staggers. It may be noted that pirouetting, swinging, and the pitching and tossing of a ship on the sea produce similar effects.

Vertigo, strictly meaning the sense of rotation, suggests dysfunction of the labyrinth or of the brain stem, whereas dizziness—the sensation of unsteadiness

—is usually due to some reduction of the blood supply to the brain, as in fainting.

Deafness

As will be understood from the preceding considerations, deafness is of two types:

(*a*) Conductive deafness—arising from obstruction to sound waves.

(*b*) Nerve deafness, the cause of which may rest in the nerve endings in the cochlea, in the auditory nerve or in the auditory cortex.

Differentiation between the two types may be difficult to achieve. The surgeon uses a tuning fork test to discover whether air-conduction is greater than bone conduction (as it should be) or vice versa. When deafness is present and the middle ear is shown to be normal by this test, the nerve type of deafness exists. Other tests are used to decide which ear is the more affected.

Accurate estimation of hearing is made by means of an electric apparatus called an audiometer. This is an apparatus by which graphs can be charted showing the degree and type of hearing loss. The record is useful for future comparison for deciding on treatment and also for the provision of a hearing aid to suit the individual patient. The use of the audiometer demands a sound-proof room. Each ear is tested separately and the test takes twenty minutes or longer. Sound is produced electrically and the patient indicates the quietest sound that can be perceived at a given pitch.

When a patient is unequally deaf in the two ears, it is necessary to distinguish the hearing in the ear being tested from sounds heard by the opposite ear. For this purpose, Barany's noise box (see page 246) is used. This contains a small hammer which can be set to vibrate against a diaphragm. An ear-piece from the box is put into the ear not being tested and the noise of the vibration will mask the sounds used for the hearing test on the opposite ear.

Hearing Aids

A great number of hearing aids have been designed, varying very much in pattern. They fall into two main groups.

1. Ear trumpets, auricles and other sound-collecting apparatus without electricity. The trumpet is the best of these, especially for elderly patients, but has the disadvantage of being conspicuous and is now used extremely rarely.

2. Electrical aids, (a) of the valve type, (b) transistors. These can be delicately adjusted to amplify sounds in accordance with the record of hearing obtained by audiometer. The varieties of electric aids differ in pattern and weight in order to suit the habits and occupation of the users. Body-level aids tend to be bulky; ear level aids are less conspicuous. In general, transistor aids are less cumbersome, less conspicuous, and give the less distorted amplification; also, batteries last longer. The valve amplifying aids last longer. If nurses are consulted, they should warn patients not to purchase an aid without consulting an otologist. "Background" noises may be very troublesome in electric aids, and adequate trial in the home and at work is to be recommended before the choice is made.

21

Diseases of the external ear

Otitis Externa

Various skin diseases affect the external ear. By far the most common of these is seborrhœic dermatitis of the scalp which produces excessive dandruff. Extreme irritation results which is worse in hot weather and is increased by bathing. This condition often also affects the back of the ears causing painful cracks at the top and bottom of the junction of the auricle with the head. Scratching causes invasion by bacteria of the skin and the meatal wall. The bacteriology is often mixed. *Ps. pyocyaneas* is commonly found. Staphylococci are secondary invaders.

Treatment.—The scalp is treated with frequent shampoos with spirit soap and the application of lotions or ointment prescribed by the skin specialist. For the ear condition meticulous toilet is essential. Treatment can only be adequately carried out by trained personnel—the patient cannot be trusted to do it. Hence, nursing is important. The meatus must be gently mopped right down to the drum under direct vision. Then the appropriate medication is applied. There may be daily packing, with, for example, 8 per cent. aluminium acetate or glycerine and ichthyol. Later, neomycin and hydrocortisone ointments are often used. (*N.B.* Antibiotics are used only with steroids.) Drops are applied when the skin is almost healed.

Eczema of the Ear

Eczema is a sensitization dermatitis characterized by the formation of vesicles which rupture and discharge a serous fluid. This exudate either dries and forms pin-head crusts, or a continuous oozing occurs. As the inflammatory reaction dies down, the exudate ceases, and the skin becomes covered with small scales. This sequence of events may last several weeks or years and the disease may be arrested for long periods.

Treatment.—As eczema is generally due to allergy (see page 78) or to chemical irritation, the patient is usually treated generally. The local treatment consists of cleanliness, the relief of irritation and the avoidance of scratching. A useful application to help in relief and healing is a paint containing gentian violet. The external meatus should be swabbed with this solution, and then dried by means of a blower.

Herpes Simplex and Herpes Zoster

Both these conditions occasionally affect the external ear and are treated as other forms of otitis externa.

Herpes zoster is an acute inflammation of the sensory ganglion of a cutaneous nerve and is characterized by groups of vesicles which last for 1 to 2 weeks and then dry, leaving scarred areas. It can occur on the 5th and 7th cranial nerves—the Gasserian and geniculate ganglia. The disease is marked by severe pain and irritation which may persist for many months after the skin lesion has healed.

Furunculosis

Boils commonly arise in the cartilaginous portion of the external auditory meatus, and like boils elsewhere (see page 64, furunculosis of the nose) arise as staphylococcal infections of the hair follicles. They are often secondary to seborrhœic dermatitis. They may develop into abscesses.

Symptoms.—There is severe pain owing to the unyielding texture of the tissues. The pain is felt in the front of the ear (as distinct from mastoid pain which is behind) which is tender on manipulation. Swelling of the meatus produces obstructive deafness. As each boil "points" and discharges its contents, there is a remission of pain, but fresh boils tend to arise.

Treatment.—Systemic treatment with penicillin and/or a sulphonamide preparation is usually commenced at the onset of the condition. The pain may be relieved to some extent by the application of heat. Where the meatus is swollen, gauze wicks soaked in warm glycerin and 10 per cent. ichthyol may be gently packed into the auditory canal and a thermal pad applied outside. For recurrent boils, vaccine therapy is sometimes used.

Aspergillosis (Otomycosis)

This is a fungoid infection which attacks the external auditory meatus. It produces a membrane looking rather like damp blotting paper covered with black or yellow spots. The patient complains of irritation and discharge.

The treatment commonly employed is the application of Nystatin or gentian violet. Oils and ointments must not be applied to the ear as these encourage the growth of the fungus.

Other fungi may cause otomycosis. Griseofulvin taken internally is now used as treatment.

Hæmatoma of the Auricle

This unsightly condition is caused by injury, particularly from a blow on the ear as in boxing. Small bruises require no treatment as a rule, but a large hæmatoma, besides being painful owing to the retention of blood in dense tissues that cannot swell easily, is in danger of becoming infected. Infection commonly leads to the destruction of cartilage.

Treatment of a Large Hæmatoma.—The pinna is first cleaned, using swabs dipped in methylated spirit. The hæmatoma is then aspirated, using a hypodermic syringe and needle, with full aseptic technique. A dressing is then firmly bandaged in position.

Alternatively, the Elastoplast technique may be employed. This consists of cleaning the ear, aspirating the blood-stained contents of the hæmatoma, filling the hollows of the pinna with a mould of Stent's compound or sponge rubber and securing this with Elastoplast. The strapping is laid on both sides of the auricle and the edges are stuck to each other. The surplus is then trimmed to make a neat dressing. This is left for 10 days. If necessary, the aspiration is repeated.

Excess of Wax in the Ear

The normal cerumen secreted in the auditory meatus occasionally accumulates in the lower corner of the meatus against the ear drum and may interfere with hearing. This usually happens in persons suffering from some degree of seborrhœic dermatitis. The mass contains flakes of epithelial debris. This is usually removed by careful syringing (see page 33). But, if the drum is known to be perforated, syringing should not be carried out, owing to the danger of fluid entering the middle ear and setting up inflammation. Instead, the wax is picked out by the doctor, using a sharp hook.

Foreign Bodies in the Ear

It is most important that amateur attempts to remove a hard foreign body from the ear should be discouraged, especially with a sharp instrument which may damage the ear drum. Owing to the curves of the external auditory meatus, it is easier to push an object into an inaccessible part of the canal than to withdraw it. Sometimes, however, an insect such as a fly or a spider may find its way into an ear, and an attempt to remove it should be made. A fly buzzing inside one's ear makes a thunderous roar, most alarming to a child and quite disturbing to an adult. A little warm water inserted into the meatus from a teaspoon may float out the insect. If this is not effective, spirit drops should be instilled to kill the insect, which is then syringed out. A vegetable object such as a pea should not be treated by syringing, because, if the procedure fails to remove it, the pea will swell, become impacted and will be more difficult to remove. Mineral objects, such as beads, can often be syringed out, but if this is unsuccessful, the surgeon will use aural forceps or a sharp hook in a strong reflected light. On rare occasions, an incision behind the auricle is necessary to remove the object.

Irritation caused by discharge sometimes explains why a child inserts foreign bodies into the ear. Obstruction of drainage may follow, giving rise to severe symptoms of sepsis.

Rupture of the Ear Drum

This may be the result of a blow over the external meatus or from bomb explosions or gunfire, or may be due to fracture of the skull. Whatever the cause, even if there is bleeding from the ear, the only treatment should be to apply a sterile gauze dressing and give an antibiotic to prevent infection. If suppuration should follow the rupture, then the patient is treated for acute otitis media (see page 212).

Exostosis of the Ear

Bony outgrowths occasionally arise from the wall of the external auditory meatus. They are usually single but may be multiple, and the bone composing them is much more dense than that of the meatus.

If large, they cause obstructive deafness, and will complicate the treatment of otitis externa. Wax may accumulate.

Removal is difficult owing to the hardness of the exostosis and its common position in the posterior meatal wall, in close relation with the facial nerve and other important structures. If operation is considered necessary, the approach may be either through the meatus or behind the ear.

New Growths of the External Ear

Rodent ulcer and squamous epitheliomata are comparatively common in the external ear. A rodent ulcer arises on the auricle; an epithelioma may develop on the concha or in the external meatus. On the concha it is of the ulcerative type; in the meatus it is sessile or papillomatous.

Treatment.—Small ulcers on the concha may be treated by excision or the application of a radium plaque. Growths in the external meatus require excision of the whole cartilaginous meatus. When the growth is near the drum, radical mastoidectomy is often advisable in order to remove a safe margin of bone and epithelium. This is usually combined with irradiation.

22

Diseases of the middle ear

Acute Otitis Media

Infection of the middle ear almost always travels from the nasopharynx via the Eustachian tube. The presence of adenoids and the wider straighter Eustachian tube of childhood both favour this passage of infection. Otitis media is particularly common after infections of the upper respiratory tract—for example, influenza, scarlet fever, measles, and diphtheria. It sometimes follows swimming in public baths, but often inflammation following such exercise is due to micro-organisms already present in the nose and throat. The organisms responsible for otitis media are the hæmolytic *Streptococcus pyogenes*, *Streptococcus viridans*, staphylococcus and pneumococci. Any infection may lead to bone destruction and intracranial complications (see page 219).

In the early stages of inflammation, the mucous membrane of the middle ear is reddened, then it exudes serous fluid which collects in the cavity. The infection spreads to the mastoid air-cells and if not released the exudate soon becomes purulent.

Signs and Symptoms.—At first, the patient notices slight deafness and popping noises in the ear. These are quickly succeeded by pain and the condition rapidly becomes worse. Pain and deafness are the prominent symptoms. There may be tinnitus (noises in the ear) of a pulsating nature but these are not usually severe. The pain is more severe at night. There may be tenderness over the mastoid process. An infant suffering from acute otitis media will be fretful and restless, rubbing his hand over his ear and his head in the pillow. The temperature is usually raised and may reach 39.5°C (103°F) or 40°C (104°F) in children. On examination, the ear drum is seen to be flushed, with a network of dilated blood vessels. At a very early stage of inflammation, the malleus is still visible. In a few

Fig. 43.—Applying a Bandage to the Ear.

hours, the membrane is bulging and bright red, and the malleus is obscured. If the inflammation is untreated, a yellow spot appears in front of or behind the handle of the malleus, rupture follows and blood-stained pus escapes into the meatus. Pain is then relieved as a rule. If it persists, the indication is probably the retention of pus in the mastoid process. The patient is often not admitted to hospital, but an increasing deafness accompanying otitis media must be regarded as a grave sign.

Treatment.—This turns upon the severity of the condition on the one hand and the stage it has reached on the other. In a mild case, the doctor may decide that all that are needed are such simple remedies as aspirin and a well-protected hot water-bottle.

Where the patient is ill and whether the drum has ruptured or not, penicillin or some other antibiotic is given. If the drum has ruptured, a sterile dressing is kept over the ear, and discharge is either mopped out or gently syringed away daily. The patient is usually kept in bed. The accompanying nasal infection is treated by steam inhalations, etc.

The operation of myringotomy (incision of the ear drum) is mainly reserved for those conditions where fluid continues to accumulate in the tympanum after adequate antibiotic treatment, where pain or where deafness persists.

The nurse's duties in relation to these patients will be to give the antibiotics and other medicines, to change the ear dressings and to report any signs of complications such as mastoiditis or intracranial invasion by the infection.

Acute Mastoiditis

This has become exceedingly rare and is usually seen in neglected cases of acute otitis media. The complication is indicated by an intensification of the symptoms. Pain becomes severe. Tenderness, and usually redness and swelling occur behind the ear. In late cases, the swelling thrusts the auricle forward in a characteristic fashion. The amount of discharge usually increases but may lessen temporarily. In infants, the bony outer wall of the mastoid is thin and may rupture, so that pus may escape and form an abscess beneath the skin.

Treatment.—Intensive antibiotic therapy may still check the infection in the early stage before breakdown of bone and abscess formation have occurred, but the patient must be kept under close observation. The operation of mastoidectomy is usually needed.

Chronic Otitis Media

The change from acute otitis to the chronic form is ill-defined, but the term "chronic suppurative otitis media" is applied when there is suppuration of long standing with no signs of acute inflammation. Pain is usually absent.

The *discharge* varies from thin mucopurulent secretion to offensive, cheesy material which escapes into the external meatus through a perforation in the drum.

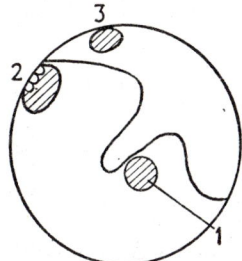

FIG. 44.—PERFORATIONS OF THE DRUM
1. Central; 2. Marginal, with granulations; 3. Attic perforation which is associated with cholesteatoma.

If scanty it may even escape the patient's notice! The odour is dependent upon secondary infection due to obstructed drainage. The nature of the discharge helps to indicate the primary source of the otitis. 1. Mucoid discharge is characteristic of a primary post-nasal infection, spreading by the Eustachian tube into the lower part of the middle ear. 2. A thick offensive discharge indicates bony disease in the attic or mastoid bone. The site of the disease is indicated by the position of the perforation. Frequently attic perforations can be seen, but in some cases the discharge is so scanty that it dries over a perforation and obscures it. In these cases, the discharge becomes foul-smelling, and cholesteatoma (see page 217) is suspected. Blood-stained discharge indicates granulation tissue and polypi which in turn point to deep-seated disease of bone.

Deafness in some degree, from slight impairment to complete absence of hearing, accompanies chronic otitis media.

Granulations are bright red, sessile masses. They bleed readily, and can be touched by a probe without producing pain. A polypus does not differ materially from granulation tissue. It is attached by a stalk and being covered with squamous epithelium, it does not bleed when touched, but it may obscure the details of the drum.

Secretory Otitis Media ("Glue Ear")

This is a condition seen with increasing frequency during recent years. A clear exudate fills the middle ear and the tympanic membrane often has a yellowish tinge. The patient complains of stuffiness in the ear. It is due to a dysfunction of the Eustachian Tube following repeated acute attacks of infection or obstruction (e.g. from adenoids) or alterations in air pressure such as occur when landing in an aircraft. In all these cases, air cannot enter the middle ear from the tube, and middle ear effusion often results.

Treatment.—In children, Politzeration (see page 23) is performed daily by nursing staff, combined with nasal decongestants. If this fails to cure the condition, surgery under a short anæsthetic is required (see myringotomy and insertion of grommets, page 233). For adults, Politzerization may be effective; more often, Eustachian catheterization or myringotomy with insertion of a drain is necessary. If drainage is inadequate, fibrous adhesions may bind the ossicles,

DISEASES OF THE MIDDLE EAR

retracting the tympanic membrane and causing conductive or adhesive deafness and eventually cholesteatoma formation. In severe cases, this leads to the necessity for a hearing aid.

Cholesteatoma

This is a yellowish-grey mass consisting of epithelial tissue, pus and crystals of cholesterin. It occurs in the middle ear and may be either the cause or the result of chronic suppuration, according to its origin. It may be formed in various ways:

(*a*) As an aberration of development, squamous epithelium being included in other tissues. This form may occur within the cranial cavity.

(*b*) As a result of inflammation, by destruction of the edge of the drum and the ingrowth of epithelium from the external meatus. Constant desquamation of epithelial cells forms a mass which erodes bone. It may destroy the whole of the middle and inner ear and even constitute an intracranial tumour. In the middle ear it is liable to keep up an infection and lead to serious intracranial complications.

(*c*) The character of the epithelium in the middle ear changes from ciliated to stratified epithelium as a result of infection.

Spread of Infection from the Middle Ear

A backward spread of infection from the middle ear will penetrate:

(*a*) The mastoid air cells. This is commonly concurrent with otitis media.

(*b*) The lateral sinus, further back.

(*c*) The cerebellum, still further back.

An inward spread will reach the inner ear, causing labyrinthitis.

An upward spread will involve the temporal lobe of

the brain, leading to meningitis, cerebral abscess and other intracranial complications.

Complications of Middle Ear Disease

All of these are becoming more rare and occur usually in acute exacerbations of chronic ear infections.

Lateral Sinus Thrombosis

Venous infection with thrombosis occurs first in a tributary vein and spreads quickly into the lateral sinus, part of which projects into the mastoid process, so that its wall easily becomes infected and adherent to the bone. This may lead to abscesses around the sinus (perisinous abscess). These are not uncommon in children. Should the sinus itself become inflamed, the very serious condition of thrombosis may develop. Particles of septic clot may be broken off into the blood stream and produce pyæmia (abscesses forming in other part of the body), or the patient may develop septicæmia.

Signs.—Sinus thrombosis follows two main types:

(*a*) The acute fulminating type which is typically shown by rigors, or convulsions in infancy, and a persistently swinging temperature.

(*b*) The commoner form in which the ear continues to discharge and there are unexplained spikes of pyrexia. The infection occasionally spreads down the jugular vein. The sternomastoid muscle is painful and tender. The patient is well orientated and there is no headache unless the infection spreads to the meninges.

Diagnosis of thrombosis is made by Queckenstedt's test. For this purpose a lumbar puncture is performed, and the jugular vein on the affected side is compressed. If this causes no rise of pressure in the spinal fluid, obstruction is present at a higher level.

Treatment.—The ear condition will probably indicate the need for a mastoid operation. When this has been

DISEASES OF THE MIDDLE EAR

completed the bone over the sinus (if not destroyed by the disease) is removed, the lateral sinus is incised and the clot removed. Bleeding is controlled by the insertion of gauze packing between the sinus and the bone.

In dressing the mastoid wound, the gauze packing (unless of the absorbable variety) should be removed gradually, an inch or so each day, in order to avoid bleeding, which would probably occur should the packing be removed suddenly.

Antibiotics should be continued until after the symptoms have subsided.

Intracranial Complications of Otitis

By means of septic thrombi carried in the blood stream, infection from the middle or inner ear can spread into the cranium. It may pass directly through the thin bone which forms the roof of the middle ear, or through the petrous bone or through anatomical channels between the ear and the brain, for example, through the labyrinth by the internal auditory meatus. A diffuse meningitis may follow, or the infection may be localized into an abscess. The abscess may be between the dura and the bone (extradural) or within the dura (subdural) or in the brain substance itself.

Meningitis

Signs and Symptoms.—With the onset of meningitis fever becomes higher, there is restlessness and loss of appetite. Meningeal irritation is first shown by discomfort on flexing the head forward and photophobia with generalized headache. This is followed by severe headache and rigidity of the neck. There are increased deep reflexes and characteristic changes in the cerebrospinal fluid—notably a decrease in carbohydrate, and an increased cell count. Bacteria may be grown by culture of the fluid. As the intracranial pressure rises, other symptoms appear, such as vomiting, insomnia, a relatively slow pulse rate and Cheyne-Stokes respiration. The patient lies on his back with his eyes closed, in a stupor from which he may be easily roused.

The diagnosis is established by lumbar puncture, and this should be done on the earliest suspicion of meningitis. The meningitis complicating otitis media is usually due to the streptococcus, the staphylococcus or the pneumococcus. The last was once considered the most serious but the prognosis has been improved by sulpha therapy. Nowadays the most dangerous infections are those that are less sensitive to antibiotics and the sulpha drugs, for example, *Proteus vulgaris* (varieties of which are commonly responsible for epidemic enteritis) and *Hæmophilus influenzæ*. Sulpha preparations find their way into the cerebrospinal fluid. Penicillin does not.

Treatment.—When the causative organism is found, the appropriate preparation is given. Sulpha drugs are given in full doses orally (or intravenously if there is vomiting). Penicillin is given intramuscularly or intravenously. Free drainage of the primary source of infection is combined with repeated lumbar puncture. Dehydration must be avoided and intravenous fluid is often required. A patient with meningitis is very ill and needs much patience and attention from his nurses, together with careful observation and recording of all vital signs. He may be irrational, irritable or delirious and the nurse will need all her tact to carry out the necessary care of mouth, pressure areas, and feeding. A sedative is often given before attempting lumbar puncture.

Intracranial Abscesses

Extradural Abscess, rarely diagnosed before operation as it is part of a mastoid abscess, gives no special symptoms beyond those of mastoid infection. Necrosis of bone in the mastoid area reaches the middle, or sometimes the posterior cranial fossa, where the dura mater reacts by thickening and closing off the infection. Unless the abscess is drained, the infection may penetrate the dura mater and other meninges, causing first a stage of encephalitis and then abscess of the brain tissue.

Cerebral Abscess is most commonly situated in the temporal lobe. The mode of spread is usually by a septic thrombophlebitis. The abscess is at first thin-walled and poorly shut off; later, it becomes thick-walled.

Symptoms.—Headache, vomiting, giddiness and slowness of speech and thought are the general symptoms. In the early stages, the temperature and pulse rates may be raised in response to the sepsis, but as the compression of the brain increases, the temperature becomes subnormal and the pulse slow. Weakness of certain muscles may indicate to the doctor the position of the abscess. Lumbar puncture is performed only with the greatest caution lest sudden alteration in pressure cause harm. If the cerebrospinal fluid is examined it is found to have fewer chlorides and more protein than normal. Should the abscess be leaking into the ventricles or the subarachnoid space, the fluid will be turbid.

An abscess in the left temporal lobe of a right-handed patient produces aphasia—the inability to name common objects although the patient can describe them.

Eye changes may accompany cerebral abscess.

Cerebellar Abscess in the posterior cranial fossa causes symptoms of cerebral infection and raised intracranial pressure as previously described. The localizing symptoms are a varying nystagmus (oscillation of the eyeball) and loss of muscular co-ordination.

Treatment of Brain Abscess.—The nursing treatment is very important as the patient may be unconscious or disorientated and may be incontinent. He may need nasal feeding or intravenous therapy. The diagnostic treatment will be lumbar puncture, and encephalography or arteriography. Surgical treatment is carried out by a neurosurgeon. Generally burr holes are made, the abscess is tapped and the cavity is filled with antibiotic. This is repeated whenever signs of raised intracranial pressure occur again until the abscess has contracted to a small unimportant scar. The abscess may be dissected out if it fails to contract satisfactorily.

The primary ear condition is treated when the neurosurgeon thinks the patient is fit for this.

Facial Paralysis of Otitic Origin

The facial nerve may be involved by an infection of the mastoid bone cells surrounding the facial canal, or may be damaged during operation.

As the facial nerve supplies the muscles of expression, complete paralysis is shown by marked asymmetry of the face, the affected side being devoid of its natural folds and expression. Any attempt at smiling causes the face to be drawn to the opposite side. The patient cannot raise the eyebrow or close the eye or show his teeth on the paralysed side. He cannot whistle or pronounce the labial consonants. Paralysis of the buccinator muscle allows food to collect between the gum and the cheek. The chorda tympani branch of the facial nerve may be damaged, resulting in loss of taste and a diminished salivary secretion.

Facial paralysis also occurs without apparent cause and without ear disease. These ideopathic types are known as Bell's palsy.

Treatment: (a) *Before operation.* If signs of facial paralysis appear early in the course of an acute middle ear infection, they will usually disappear with antibiotic treatment. In the established case of otitis media, operation and decompression of the nerve via the mastoid is usually needed.

(*b*) *During operation.* Should the nerve be damaged during operation, it is immediately sutured.

(*c*) *After operation.* If the paralysis is noticed soon after operation, but is incomplete, recovery is likely. If it is complete, the operation cavity will probably need to be reopened and the nerve explored. If the paralysis develops a few days after operation, it will almost certainly recover.

After section of the nerve and grafting, recovery usually takes about 12 months, and then the movements of the facial muscles are not perfect. The patient is usually provided with a splint to raise the corner of the mouth and so avoid over-stretching the cheek muscles. Especial care must be taken to ensure oral cleanliness as the patient cannot wash out the mouth on the affected side. Since normal blinking does not occur on the affected side, the nurse should bathe the eye carefully. Sometimes the eyelids may need suturing to protect the cornea (tarsorrhaphy).

(*d*) *Bell's palsy* usually responds to physiotherapy, but in certain circumstances the nerve may need to be decompressed as it lies in its bony canal in order to promote recovery.

Otosclerosis

This is a disease affecting the middle and inner ear and is at present of unknown origin. It causes progressive conductive deafness, commencing in youth. Females suffer more often than males, and there is a familial tendency. For some reason, perhaps metabolic, normal bone in the labyrinth is absorbed and a deposit of new vascular web-like bone appears in its place. There is usually more than one primary focus. The area around the oval window is most often first affected, less frequently the round window, but the condition slowly spreads through the labyrinth. In time this spongy bone becomes compact. Deafness occurs as soon as the windows cease to vibrate normally, and increases as the stapes becomes fixed. The patient commonly hears much better in a noise. She speaks in a typically soft voice, in contrast with the loud voice of a person with nerve deafness.

On examination, the ear drum appears normal. Tuning fork tests show a conductive deafness and, in older patients, some nerve deafness. There is no improvement in hearing after inflation of the Eustachian tube, which is dry and clear.

Treatment.—This is usually surgical. The stapes is removed completely and replaced by a prosthesis. Hearing aids can be supplied if the patient is elderly or does not wish for operation or if there is too much internal ear damage.

23

Diseases of the inner ear

Disease of the inner ear produces dizziness due to disturbance of the fluid levels in the semicircular canals of the labyrinth or of the function of the auditory nerve, or both. Deafness resulting from disease of the inner ear occurs in varying degrees but hearing is never completely lost unless the cochlea or the auditory nerve is destroyed.

Inner Ear Deafness

Inner ear deafness may be congenital, or acquired.

Causes of Congenital Inner Ear Deafness

1. Maldevelopment of the ear. Essential parts may be absent.
2. Congenital syphilis.
3. Disease of the mother during pregnancy. Rubella (German measles) particularly is held responsible for defect in the cochlear mechanism.
4. The taking of quinine by the pregnant woman.
5. Rhesus factor antibodies in the mother's blood.

Causes of Acquired Inner Ear Deafness

1. Labyrinthitis. This may be a non-suppurative effusion, usually in one ear only, following mumps. Cerebrospinal meningitis may cause bilateral inflammation of the labyrinth which is often permanent.
2. Concussion. A blow or explosion without obvious injury to the structure of the ear may cause destruction of the auditory nerve endings.
3. Occupation. Exposure to percussive noises as with boiler-makers or anti-aircraft gunners may result

in permanent damage to hearing. It can be prevented by the wearing of a well-fitting helmet. Flying men may be provided with ear plugs.

4. Old age. Senile deafness is due to the degeneration of the auditory nerve. There is often an atrophy of part of the membranous cochlea causing loss of hearing for high notes. The deafness is usually bilateral and is not accompanied by tinnitus.

Deafness in Infancy

This condition may be inherited or congenital, due to maldevelopment or intra-uterine disease affecting the ear, but deafness may be acquired at a very early age, as from meningitis and this will prevent the child from learning to speak. The child requires careful training in lip reading and a transistor hearing aid. The latter may be supplied to babies in cots, and their early use can lead to accurate development of speech. If the hearing loss is severe, special educational methods will be needed.

Tests of Vestibular Function

Disease of the vestibule causes three main symptoms:
1. Vertigo.
2. Nausea and vomiting—these are called "visceral reflexes".
3. Nystagmus.

Tests are used to stimulate the labyrinth in various ways, comparisons being made between the reactions of the two ears in order to discover the presence of abnormality. The common tests are the Caloric Test and the Rotation Test.

The Caloric Test.—This depends on convection currents produced in the semicircular canals by heating or cooling a portion of the labyrinth. The flow of endolymph stimulates specialized nerve endings causing giddiness and nystagmus. Since cold produces a

DISEASES OF THE INNER EAR

greater response than heat, cold water is used first. If the drum is perforated, air may be introduced instead of water.

The apparatus required is a 1 litre douche can with about 1½ metres of rubber tubing, ending in a nozzle and controlled by a pinch clip, a thermometer and mixer, a receiver, and a stop-watch.

FIG. 45.—THE CALORIC TEST.
The nurse's hands are shown holding the tube in the meatus and steadying the dish. A thermometer and mixer stand on a nearby table.

The patient lies on his back, and his head is raised 30°, which brings his lateral semicircular canals into the vertical position. A stand or shelf holds the douche can approximately 61 cm above the ears. The can is filled with water at 30°C (86°F), i.e. 7°C below body temperature, the temperature being measured by a thermometer and the water well mixed. The nurse runs a little water through the tubing, pinches the rubber tubing and hands the nozzle to the doctor, who places it in the patient's left ear and tells him to fix his eyes on a certain spot. The nurse then holds the nozzle in the meatus and steadies the kidney dish below it. The doctor holds the stop-watch and gives word for the irrigation to begin. After exactly 40 seconds, the nurse is told to stop the flow, while the doctor watches the patient's eyes for nystagmus. The moment this ceases, he stops the watch and records the duration. After a pause of 5 minutes to allow the labyrinth to recover from the stimulation, the right ear is tested in the same way. Water at 44°C (111°F), i.e. 7°C above body temperature, is then used on first the left, then the right ear, waiting 5 minutes between each test. If no nystagmus occurs, a further test using water at 20°C, or 68°F, is used. The normal duration of the nystagmus is 2 minutes for each reading. With loss of function, it is less than this.

The Rotation Test.—The patient sits in a rotating chair. Rotation of the chair with the patient holding his head in varying positions will produce nystagmus of varying character and duration. Both ears are affected at the same time but in opposite directions. The correct interpretation of the test is difficult. The tendency to fall is away from the affected labyrinth, but the patient may make such an effort to recover that he falls the other way.

The duration of the nystagmus is noted in seconds. If no nystagmus is produced, the labyrinth is assumed to be functionless.

More accurate methods are involved in what is called Electronystagmography. This allows accurate measurement of the speed, amplitude and frequency of the nystagmus; these measurements can be more important than duration.

Aural Vertigo

As has been mentioned before, dizziness may occur in a large number of conditions concerned with the cardiovascular system. Vertigo whose origin is in the ear itself may be due to:

Obstruction of the Eustachian canal.
Middle ear disease.
} Disturbance of pressure in the middle ear may affect the labyrinth.

Labyrinthitis: aural vertigo with suppuration.

Ménière's disease: a non-suppurative condition of the labyrinth causing paroxysmal attacks of vertigo.

Tumour in the course of the eighth nerve, for example, a temporal lobe tumour or a cerebellar tumour.

It may also occur after stapedectomy and other ear operations for a few days.

Suppurative Labyrinthitis

Suppurative labyrinthitis may follow otitis media or an injury to the ear. Circumscribed and diffuse types are described but the difference is only one of degree. It usually follows chronic otitis media which is frequently due to cholesteatoma.

Symptoms.—These are giddiness, especially on turning quickly or bending, loss of balance, nausea and vomiting. Nystagmus is present. On applying the caloric test a diminished reaction is found in the affected ear. Hearing is fairly good as a rule, although it may fade, or the patient may be deaf from the original disease. If a fistula from the middle ear is present, then any sudden change in middle ear pressure will immediately produce acute labyrinthine reactions, provided that the labyrinth is functioning. The test is to exert sudden pressure on the tragus or to insert the nozzle of a Politzer bag into the external auditory meatus and apply suction or pressure.

Treatment.—The patient should be kept quietly at rest in bed until symptoms have settled, penicillin or sulphonamide therapy being administered. When the symptoms have subsided, a mastoidectomy is performed. If there is total loss of hearing, it is wise to open the labyrinth. It may contain pus. Careful watch must always be made for meningitis.

Positional Vertigo

The patient only feels giddy when his head is put in a certain position. If he is seen during an attack, nystagmus will be noticed. Occasionally there is nausea but there is no increase in deafness. The condition is usually due to a disturbance in the otolith apparatus of the semicircular canals and is self-limiting. The patient is often anxious and a tranquillizing drug may be prescribed.

Ménière's Disease (Paroxysmal Aural Vertigo)

This is a non-suppurative condition in which there is a hydrops distension of the membranous labyrinth, characterized by sudden vertigo in recurrent attacks associated with deafness and tinnitus. The deafness is very often pre-existent. It is perceptive and the caloric test shows diminished labyrinthine function.

Symptoms.—The suddenness of the vertigo is the distinguishing feature of the condition. It may occur at night and waken the patient. Both ears may be affected. The giddiness is rotatory and, as a rule, in a definite direction. Both tinnitus and deafness are worse during the attack. As attacks become more frequent, deafness tends to persist and may become complete. Nystagmus is present during the paroxysms, but the patient's distress prevents full examination. The patient is quite helpless and incapacitated by the vertigo which may last a number of hours or days, and then passes off completely. At first, the attacks occur at long intervals and are comparatively slight, but their severity increases with their recurrence.

DISEASES OF THE INNER EAR

Treatment.—In the acute attack, sodium phenobarbitone 60 mg to 200 mg, or Largactil is given by injection. It is of the utmost importance to reassure the patient that improvement will be achieved. He can be told that he is suffering from a definite disease —not "merely from nerves". The fear of an attack during traffic or work is liable to make him lose self-confidence and the nurse can do a great deal to improve his morale. The underlying cause of the attacks can be explained to most patients.

In the established case, a sedative such as 30 mg of phenobarbitone is given three times a day. Nicotinic acid up to 300 mg daily and restricted salt and fluid help control most patients satisfactorily. However, relapses are common.

Should dietetic and sedative treatment not be effective, an operation may be decided upon. The labyrinth on the affected side may be destroyed in various ways. The power of compensation in a labyrinthine mechanism is very great. If one is destroyed, the surviving labyrinth assumes control, and in a few weeks, giddiness ceases. Any hearing that the patient may have had in that ear is lost.

Recently, the use of ultrasound directed selectively at the semicircular canals of the affected side has been used. This is done via a Schwartze mastoid approach using special apparatus. The pre-operative hearing is usually retained.

Vestibular Neuronitis

This type of vertigo occurs in younger patients than does Ménière's disease. It is probably consequent on infective conditions of the nose and throat or may be caused by a virus infection. The nature of the attack is similar to Ménière's disease. Recurrent attacks are unlikely. Antihistamine drugs are helpful in its control.

Acoustic Neuroma

This is a neurofibroma of the auditory nerve. The symptoms are similar to Ménière's disease so that diagnosis is not an easy matter. The otologist will usually refer the patient to a neurosurgeon for treatment.

24

Operations on the ear

Pre-operative Treatment

Ear operations in this country are nearly always performed under general anæsthesia. The local preparation requires the shaving of the head and neck for about 5 cm around the auricle. The remaining hair may be washed and must be fastened securely away from the operation site. If the operation is for treatment of acute infection, the patient has a considerable amount of tenderness and the shaving is occasionally done after the patient is anæsthetized. If not, it must be done gently, care being taken that the razor blade is sharp. The pinna and the meatus should be mopped clean and may be syringed. The skin is cleaned with spirit and perhaps some antiseptic of the surgeon's choice.

Myringotomy

This minor operation is carried out for acute otitis or for secretory otitis media (page 216). If need be, it is done under general anæsthesia through an aural speculum. More often it is an Out-Patient procedure carried out without anæsthetic for painless catarrhal otitis. In each case, a curved incision is made in the drum by means of a bayonet-shaped myringotome. In acute conditions an immediate escape of discharge follows, and this is mopped away with a gauze strip. A swab is sent to the laboratory to discover the organisms present and their sensitivity. After operation the ear should be inspected frequently to ensure that the opening is adequate and the drainage free.

In secretory otitis, the discharge does not escape. As much as possible is removed by suction and a Teflon tube drain or 1 or 2 grommets (see Glossary of Instruments) are inserted.

Schwartze's Operation or Cortical Mastoidectomy

Here a curved incision is made approximately 1.3 cm behind the the auricular groove and is carried down to the bone, exposing the tip of the mastoid process. The mastoid cells and antrum are then removed with a gouge or dental burr. In the past, it has been common to leave the cavity wide open and allow it to granulate, but since the advent of sulpha and penicillin, the wound is usually stitched and drained. The drain is removed in 48 hours, the stitches in 5 days.

Radical Mastoidectomy for Chronic Disease of the Ear

By this operation the middle ear and the mastoid antrum are converted into a single cavity, two ossicles and part of the external auditory canal being removed. The posterior superior wall of the attic is removed, and any remnants that there be of the malleus and the incus. The cavity is curetted and made smooth, and all loose pieces of bone are washed out. Care is taken to avoid the lateral sinus, the facial nerve and the semicircular canals, also dislocation of the stapes, as this would open up a path into the labyrinth, into which infection might travel. The meatus is enlarged by means of specially designed flaps and the cavity is packed lightly with, for example, calcium alginate and penicillin or ribbon gauze soaked in bismuth, iodoform and paraffin paste (BIPP). As a rule, the post-auricular wound is sutured.

In some cases, after 7 to 10 days the cavity in the bone is covered with a skin graft taken from behind the ear.

Modified Radical Mastoidectomy.—The postero-superior wall of the external auditory meatus is resected, but an attempt is made to conserve as much of the drum and the ossicles as possible. The wound drains through the meatus.

OPERATIONS ON THE EAR

Tympanoplasty.—Between the cortical and radical operations there are now a whole range of operations designed to eradicate chronic disease in the middle ear and mastoid, while at the same time reconstructing a more or less effective sound-conducting mechanism. They are sometimes done end-aurally (see below) or from behind. Important principles are to put some form of graft in connection with the ossicles and to close the perforation in the drum membrane. Temporalis fascia is generally used.

This work is carried out under a Zeiss operating microscope. It will be one of the duties of the theatre nurse to familiarize herself with this instrument and to be able to adjust it.

End-aural Operations

Of recent years, operations using a different approach to the ear have been performed. Instead of using a post-

FIG. 46.—POST-AURICULAR INCISION.

auricular incision (see Fig. 46), these operations enter the ear through an incision in front of the ear through the concha into the meatus (see Fig. 47). By using this route, exostoses of the external auditory meatus may be removed without damaging the healthy mastoid process, and in certain cases, a mastoidectomy for treatment of infection can be more satisfactorily performed. Pathological tissue can be clearly seen and removed.

Pre-operative Care.—see page 233. An antibiotic course is commenced the day before operation.

Post-operative Treatment

The patient is nursed in the most comfortable position. He may get up as soon as he is able. Dramamine 25 mg is given as necessary to allay giddiness. Antibiotic therapy is continued for a 5-day course. Any pack is removed on the 1st day and any drainage tubes on the

Fig. 47.—End-aural Incision.

2nd day. The dressing is changed and the sutures removed on the 5th day. The patient may go home after this, but should wear an ear pad and bandage. He should attend the Out-Patient Department on the 10th day and then at weekly intervals. It is important for

The Surgery of Otosclerotic Deafness

Stapes Mobilization

This is done under local or general anæsthesia, via a speculum and under a microscope. The drum is reflected, the stapes is exposed and gently rocked so as to mobilize it and re-establish the vibration of the oval window.

Stapedectomy

Usually the mobilization fails. In such a case, the stapes is deliberately dislocated and its crura fractured. The oval window is re-established by removal of bone and an artificial stapes is inserted. This consists either of a fat graft on a stainless steel wire, or alternatively of a very small stainless steel or plastic piston clamped to the incus. The drum is replaced and the ear packed for a day.

The advantages of these two operations are the use of local anæsthetic, the short stay in hospital and the ultimately normal ear passage.

The results of stapedectomy are excellent and generally only limited by the efficiency of the cochlea.

Post-operative Treatment

This is as for Tympanoplasty, but the patient is nursed on the unaffected side for 24 hours. After 48 hours he may sit out of bed for a few minutes, but care must be taken as the power of balance may take some time to recover. When this is satisfactory, he is allowed home. There may be some loss of taste on one side, but this is transient. Patients are told not to blow their nose sharply.

Labyrinthectomy for Ménierè's Disease

After opening the mastoid antrum and exposing the horizontal semicircular canal, the bony wall is burred out. Thereafter, the membranous canal is deliberately picked up with a fine hook and destroyed. Inasmuch as the middle ear is not opened, the cavity can be closed, and healing occurs by first intention. The patient's vertigo is usually cured, but any residual hearing in that ear is sacrificed.

The after-treatment follows closely that of stapedectomy. The patient should be warned that a slight residual dizziness will persist for some days after operation. Usually he is allowed out of bed within a week and is given special head exercises. He may be discharged in 2 to 3 weeks and return to work in 2 months.

Alternatively the membranous labyrinth can be reached with a permeatal approach to the oval window as in stapedectomy. The membrane is again picked out on a hook and alcohol is injected.

It is very important that all post-operative dressings be performed aseptically, either in the ward, a special dressing room or in the theatre.

Appendix

GLOSSARY OF INSTRUMENTS

1. Forehead Mirror.

2. Jobson-Horne's Probe.

3. Lack's Tongue Depressor.

4. "Chiron" Clear Focus Headlight

5. Aural Specula.

6. Nasal Speculum

7. Siegl's Speculum.

8. Tuning Forks.

9. Aural Angular Dressing Forceps.

10. Laryngeal Mirrors.

11. Post nasal Mirror.

13. NASAL OR AURAL DRESSING FORCEPS. (TILLY'S)

2. EUSTACHIAN CATHETER.

14. AURISCOPE.

15. Hovell's Cautery Handle.

16. Points for Galvano-Cautery Handle.

17. Antrum Cannula.

244

18. Politzer Bag.

19. Auscultation Tube.

20. Barany's Noise Box.

21. Aural Syringe.

22. Rogers's Spray.

23. Lichtwitz's Antrum Trocar.

24. Luc's Forceps.   25. Nasal Punch Forceps (Grunwald's).

26. Heath's Guillotine.

27. Davis's Split-Blade Gag.

29. Single-Hook Retractor.
31. Double-Hook Retractor.
32. Myringotome.
28. Adenoid Curette.
30. Tracheal Hook.

33. ZEISS OPERATING MICROSCOPE.

34. Durham's Tracheostomy Cannula with Lobster-Tailed Inner Tube and Pilot.

35. "Jumbo" Size Durham's Tracheostomy Tube.

36. Bowlby's Tracheal Dilators.

37. Jackson's Tracheostomy Tube.

38. Baker's Plastic Tracheostomy Tube.

39. Negus's Œsophageal Speculum.

40. Negus's Laryngoscope.

⅓ So.

FULL SIZE

41. Specimen Œsophageal (Biopsy) Forceps.

½ Sc.

42. Harvey and Negus's Plastic Bobbins for dilation of Œsophageal Stricture.

43. Audiometer.

44. Negus's Œsophagoscope, showing Detachable Suction Tube used with it.

45. McGee's Wire-Bending Forceps.

46. Shepard's Teflon Grommet Drain Tube.

47. Schuknecht Gelfoam Wire Stapedectomy Prosthesis.

48. Shea's Stapes Replacement Strut, Polyethylene.

49. Shea's Incus Grip Strut, Teflon.

50. Shea's Teflon Piston.

51. McGee's Piston.

52. Handle of a Pistol Cautery

INDEX

Abscess: cerebellar, 221; cerebral, 218, 221; extradural, 219, 220; lung, 135; mastoid, 21, 214; of septum, 74; perisinus, 218; peritonsillar, 112; retropharyngeal, 113, 114; subdural, 219
Accessory air sinuses, 1, 2, 4, 60–63; *see also* Paranasal sinuses
Achalasia, 181
Acne rosacea, 62
Acoustic neuroma, 232
Actinomycosis, 124
Adenitis, 9, 112
Adenoidectomy, 106, 127; breathing exercises after, 136
Adenoid facies, 18
Adenoids: 5, 104, 122; bleeding, 133
Agranulocytic angina, 120
Agranulocytosis, 43, 120
Air swallowing, 169, 172
Alevaire, 145
Allergy, 78
Ampulla, 194
Anæsthesia: Caldwell-Luc operation, 93; larynx, 154, 168, 177; local, 39–40; nasal, operations, 87; tonsillectomy, 128–31; racheostomy, 161
Angina: agranulocytic, 120; Vincent's, 117
Angioma: larynx, 157; nose, 68
Angioneurotic œdema, 148
Anoxæmia, 103, 155
Antibiotics, 43–46
Antihistamine drugs, 78–79
Antimetabolite, 47
Antral window, 93
Antrostomy: intranasal, 91; radical, 93
Antrotomy, 91
Antrum: cannula, 37–38, 244; irrigation, 37; mastoid, 192, 218, 228; maxillary, 86; puncture, 91
Antrum of Highmore, *see* Maxillary sinus
Aphasia, 221
Aryepiglottic fold, 158
Arytenoid cartilages, 3, 139–41, 151
Aspergillosis, 208
Aspergillus, 21
Asphyxia, 40, 131, 155, 160, 166
Asthma, 78
Atelectasis, 135, 166
Atresia choanæ, 80
Atrophic rhinitis, 77
Attic, ear, 193, 234; perforation, 215
Audiometer, 204, 254
Auditory: nerve, 187, 201, 204, 225, 226, 232; ossicles, 192, 201, 234, 235
Auditory meatus: external, 187, 199, 207–9, 215, 229, 234, 236; internal, 197, 219
Auricle, 23, 187–88, 206, 208, 233, *see also* Ear
Auriscope, 22, 23, 243
Auscultation tube, 16, 24, 245

Balance, physiology of, 202
Barany's box, 204, 246
Bell's palsy, 222, 223
Boils: ear, 207; nose, 64, 66
Breathing: exercises, 135 habits, 4
Bronchoscope, 255
Bronchoscopy, 135, 177, 179
Burns, œsophageal, 183

Cæsium, 48
Caldwell-Luc operation, 83, 93–95, 98

257

INDEX

Caloric test, 226, 227, 229
Candida albicans, 21, 109, 119
Cardiospasm, 181
Carotid artery, ligation, 72
Catarrhal: rhinitis, 75; otitis, 233
Cauterization, nose, 72, 79, 80, 90; instruments, 244, 256
Cavernous sinus, 55, 62, 65; thrombosis, 66, 85
Cervical glands, 59, 115, 117
Chancre, tonsil, 119
Chemotherapy, 42
Children: acute laryngitis, 145; examination, 18, 19; general anæsthetic, 129; nocturnal dyspnœa, 147; obstruction of larynx, 155; preparation for hospital, 127
Chloramphenicol, 45
Choanal atresia, 80
Cholesteatoma, 215, 217, 229
Cilia, 3, 4
Cleaning of instruments, 17
Cloxacillin sodium, 44
Cobalt, 48
Cocaine, 39–41, 177
Cochlea, 191, 194–96; nerve, 197, 225
Cold, common, 6, 7, 75
Collapse, partial lung, 135
Concha, ear, 188, 211
Conchæ, nasal, 2, 58; *see* Turbinate bones
Congenital deafness, 225
Corti, organ of, 196, 199, 200
Corynebacterium diphtheriæ, 8, 80, 108, 115
Coryza, 75
Cough, 135, 144, 146, 156, 175; reflex, 41, 130, 147, 180; whooping, 13, 45
Cribriform plate, 56, 59
Cricoid cartilage, 104, 138, 139, 142
Cross-infection, 11
Croup, 145
Croupaire tent, 145
Crypts, tonsillar, 106, 108
Cut throat, 154
Cyanosis, post-operative, 103
Cytotoxic drugs, 46

Dakin syringe, 30
Deafness, 21, 199, 202, 204, 214, 223; congenital, 225; in infancy, 226
Dermatitis: auricle, 206; nose, 64
Deviation of septum, 7, 72–73, 77
Diphtheria: faucial, 115; laryngeal, 146; nasal, 80
Diverticulum, œsophageal, 182
Dohlman's operation, 183
Droplet infection, 6, 8
Dysphagia, 159, 182, 185, 186; *see also* Swallowing, difficulty
Dyspnœa, 145–48, 163, 166, 175, 176, nocturnal, 147

Ear: anatomy, 187; diseases, 206, 212, 225; drum, 21–22, 187, 190, 193, 200, 206, 209, 213, 233, 237; eczema, 206–7; examination, 21–24; exostosis, 210, 236; foreign bodies, 209; inflation, 23–24; injury 208; new growths, 211; physiology, 199–205; syringing, 33; wax, 33, 188, 209; *see also* Auricle; External ear, Inner ear; Labyrinth; Middle ear
Electronystagmography, 288
Emphysema, 175
Encephalitis, 221
End-aural operations, 235
Endoscopy, 174–80
Eosinophils in allergy, 78
Ephedrine, 26, 30
Epiglottis, 138–40, 178
Epistaxis, 70–72, 79, 87
Epithelioma: ear, 211; nose, 69
Epitympanic recess, 193
Ethmoidectomy, 95, 99
Eustachian: catheter, 24, 35, 243; tube, 104, 122, 125, 191, 200, 215, 224; *see also* Pharyngotympanic tube
Examination equipment, 16
External ear: anatomy, 187–90; diseases, 206–11

INDEX

Facial: canal, 197, 222; nerve, 197, 222; paralysis, 222
Faucial tonsil, 106–8; 122
Fibroma, larynx, 157
Fistula after antrostomy, 95
Foreign bodies: bronchus, 175; ear, 209; larynx, 156; nose, 69; œsophagus, 176; trachea, 175
Friar's balsam, 31, 89
Frontal sinuses: 60, operations, 96
Frontal sinusitis, 83
Fronto-nasal duct, 61, 96
Frostbite, 67
Fungal stomatitis (Thrush), 119
Furunculosis: ear, 207; nose, 64, 66

Gamma rays, 48
Gargles, 109
Gastroscopy, 180
Gastrotomy, 159, 186
Glandular fever, 117
Glottis, 3, 140, 145, 147, 155
Glue ear (Secretory otitis media), 216
Gold, radioactive, 48, 50
Guillotine: operation, 127; Heath's, 248

Hæmangiomata, pharynx, 124
Hæmatoma: auricle, 187, 208; nasal setptum, 74, 89
Hæmolytic streptococcus, 8, 11, 14
Hæmorrhage: carotid artery, 114; nose, 70–72
Handkerchiefs, 5, 13
Hay fever, 78
Hearing aids, 205, 224
Herpes simplex, 76
Herpes zoster, 207
Hoarseness, 144, 150, 152
Howarth's operation, 97
Hygiene: personal, 1; ward, 11
Hyoid bone, 139
Hyperbaric oxygen, 52

Hypertrophic rhinitis, 77
Hypophysectomy, 98

Immunity, 8, 13, 106
Infection: defence against, 4–8; respiratory, 6
Inflation, ear, 23–24
Influenza, 76
Inhalation, steam, 31, 83, 89
Injury: ear, 208; larynx, 154; nose, 70
Inner ear: anatomy, 193–97; diseases, 225–32
Intra-arterial infusion, 47
Intracranial complications, 218
Intranasal: antrostomy, 93; ethmoidectomy, 95
Intrinsic tumours, larynx, 158–59
Intubation, 154
Iridium, 48, 50

Jugular vein, 141, 218

Kiesselbach's area, 71
Koplik's spots, 75

Labyrinth, ear, 193–96, 224; function tests, 226–28
Labyrinthectomy, 238
Labyrinthitis, 217, 225, 229
Lacrimal duct, 2, 58 75
Laryngeal, *see* Larynx
Laryngectomy, 169–73
Laryngismus stridulus, 148
Laryngitis: acute, 144–46; chronic, 149; spasmodic, 145
Laryngofissure, 170
Laryngoscopy, 25, 156, 174, 178
Laryngostomy, 156, 168
Laryngo-tracheo-bronchitis, 145
Larynx: anæsthesia, 154; anatomy, 137; cartilages, 137–39; diphtheria, 146, examination, 24–25; foreign bodies, 156; injuries, 154; obstruction, 155; paralysis, 153; perichondritis, 154;

INDEX

Larynx—*continued*
polypi, 151; spasm, 145; syphilis, 152; tuberculosis, 151; tumours, 156–59
Lateral sinus thrombosis, 218
Leukæmia, 121
Lichtwitz trocar, 91, 247
Little's area, 71
Lung, partial collapse, 135
Lupus: erythematosus, 67; vulgaris, 66

Malignant disease: ear, 211; larynx, 157; nose, 69; œsophagus, 185
Mastoid: antrum (air cells), 192, 198, 217, 231, 234; process, 85, 192, 198, 212, 234
Mastoidectomy, 211, 215, 233, 234
Mastoiditis, 214
Maw's inhaler, 32
Maxillary sinus, 60, 61, 82, 83; infection, 82, 83; operation, 91–95
Measles, 13, 75; German, 225
Membranous labyrinth, 193, 195–97, 238
Ménière's disease, 203, 230; operation, 238
Meningitis, 218, 219, 225
Methicillin sodium, 44
Methotrexate, 47
Middle ear: anatomy, 190–93; diseases, 212–24
Mononucleosis, 117
Mucocele, 84
Mucous membrane, 2–4, 8, 56, 60, 75, 77–81, 83, 88, 94, 105, 108, 137, 139, 149, 191, 212; olfactory, 59
Mustines, 47
Myringotomy, 214, 233

Nasal, *see* Nose
Nasopharynx, 2, 104, 106, 125, 130
Negus's operation, 97
Nelson's inhaler, 32

Neomycin, 46, 206
Nephritis, after tonsillitis, 109, 111
Nerve: auditory, 183, 197, 225, 232; deafness, 204; facial, 197, 222, 234; olfactory, 56, 59; trigeminal, 54, 60, 188
Neuromuscular disorders, œsophagus, 181
Nitrogen mustard, 47
Noise, 201–2
Nose: anatomy, 53–60; bleeding, 70; broken, 70; cauterization, 72, 79, 80, 90; cavity, 2, 55–62; diseases, 64, 72–75; examination, 19; obstruction, 73, 78–81; papilloma, 68; polypi, 79, 90; swab taking, 20; *see also* Septum
Nystagmus, 221, 226–30

Obliteration, frontal sinus, 97
Œdema: glottis, 3, 109; larynx, 145, 156; angioneurotic, 148
Œsophagoscopy, 179
Œsophagus, 104, 139, 142, 173, 176; diseases, 181
Œstrogen, 78
Olfactory mucous membrane, 59
Operations: preparations, nasal, 87; *see specific terms*
Organ of Corti, 196, 198, 200, 202
Oropharynx, 104
Ossicles, auditory, 192, 234
Osteomyelitis, frontal bone, 97
Osteoplastic operation, 97
Otitis externa, 206
Otitis media, 21, 212; chronic, 215; intracranial complications, 219; secretory, 216; suppurative, 215
Otomycosis, 208
Otosclerosis, 223
Ozœna, 77

Palatine tonsils, 102
Papilloma: larynx, 156; nose, 68

INDEX

Paralysis: after diphtheria, 116; facial 198, 222; laryngeal, 153; soft palate, 116
Paranasal sinuses, 53–63; 82–85; operations, 87; tumours, 86
Paroxysmal aural vertigo, 230
Paul-Bunnel test, 117
Perichondritis, laryngeal, 151, 152, 154
Perilymph, 195, 200, 201
Peritonsillar abscess (Quinsy), 112
Pharyngeal pouch, 182
Pharyngitis: acute, 111; chronic, 123; syphilitic, 123; tuberculous, 123
Pharyngolaryngectomy, 172
Pharyngostomy, 173
Pharyngotympanic tube, 2, 23, 24, 104, 189–92
Pharynx: anatomy, 104; diseases, 111–24
Pillars of fauces, 104
Piriform fossa, 128, 138, 158
Pistons, 256
Pituitary gland removal, 98
Politzer's: bag, 229, 245; method, 23
Polymyxin, 46
Polypi: ear, 216; larynx, 151; maxillary sinus, 95; nose, 70, 90
Posterior nares, 56
Preparations, nasal operation, 87
Proetz syringe, 30
Proof puncture, maxillary antrum, 91

Queckenstedt's test, 218
Quinsy, 112

Radiotherapy, 48–51, 69, 125–26, 158, 211
Ray fungus, 124
Reissner, membrane, 200
Respiratory infections, 6–9
Rhinitis: acute, 75; allergic, 78; chronic, 77; membranous (nasal diphtheria), 80

Rhinoscopy, 33
Rhinotomy, 98
Rogers's spray, 17, 33, 246
Rotation tests, 226, 228
Rupture, eardrum, 210, 213, 214

Saccule, ear, 195, 203
Sarcoma, tonsil, 125
Scarlet fever (Scarlatina), 75, 112
Schwartze's operation, 234
Seborrhœic dermatitis, 206, 207, 209
Secretory otitis media (Glue ear), 216
Semicircular canals, 194, 195, 203, 225–27, 238
Septum: abscess, 74; anatomy, 2, 53, 57, 59; deviation, 7, 72–73, 77; hæmatoma, 74, 89; perforation, 75; submucous resection, 88
Serum sickness, 117
Shrapnell's membrane, 191
Siegl's speculum, 17, 23, 240
Sinuses: accessory air, 1, 2, 4, 60–63; ethmoidal, 63; frontal, 60–61; infections, 82, 83; maxillary, 60, 61, 82, 83; operations, 91–96; paranasal, 53–63, 82–85; *see also specific entries*
Sinusitis, 6, 9, 30, 82–85
Sneezing, 6, 75
Spasmodic laryngitis, 145
Speech: air swallowing, 169, 172; nasal, 136
Stapedectomy, 237
Stapes, 192, 200, 224, 234; mobilization 237
Stenosis: laryngeal, 152, 155; œsophageal, 184
Stomatitis, 119
Streptococcal sore throat, 108
Streptomycin, 45, 152
Stricture, œsophageal, 181
Stridor, 144, 147, 155; newborn, 147
Stylomastoid foramen, 198
Suction displacement, 30

Sulphonamides, 42
Swallowing, 141; difficulty, 109, 151, 181–86
Syphilis: larynx, 152; nose, 68; throat, 119, 123
Syringing ear, 21, 33

Temporal bone, 187–92, 198
Throat: cut, 154; diseases, 108–26; swab, 14, 109, 116; *see also* Tonsils
Thrombosis: cavernous sinus, 66, 85; lateral sinus, 218
Thrush, 119
Thyroid cartilage, 138
Thyrotomy, 170
Tinnitus, 201, 212, 226, 230
Tonsillectomy, 13, 127–36; position, 102
Tonsils: abscess, 112; anatomy, 104–7; chancre, 119; diseases, 108–22; enucleation, 127; palatine, 102; sarcoma, 125
Trachea, 142, 160–79
Tracheostomy, 116, 145–46, 149, 153–56; after-treatment, 163; emergency, 165; instruments, 251
Tracheotomy, 160
Trephine operation, 96
Tuberculosis: larynx, 151; nose, 79
Tumours: acoustic, 232; eighth nerve, 229; laryngeal, 156–59; paranasal, 86; pharyngeal, 124–26
Turbinate bones (nasal conchæ), 2, 58, 73
Tympanic cavity, 190

Tympanic membrane (tympanum), 21, 188, 200–1, 210; examination, 22

Ulcers: œsophageal, 185; rodent, 69, 211; tonsillar, 109, 123
Ultrasound, 231
Utricle, 196, 203
Uvula, 21, 104, 108, 112

Vaccines, 8
Valsalva's method, 23
Vasoconstriction, 26, 77
Vertigo, 203, 225–31, 238; paroxysmal aural, 230
Vestibular neuronitis, 231
Vestibular tests, 226–28
Vestibule: ear, 194; nose, 56, 59, 80, 87
Vincent's angina, 117
Viruses, 6, 43, 75, 76, 117
Vocal abuse, 149
Vocal cords, 139; nodules, 150; paralysis, 153
Voice production, 137
Vomer, 57

Waldeyer's ring, 105-6
Wax, ear, 21, 33, 188, 189, 209
Window: round, 193–95, 201; oval, 189, 191, 201, 237, 238

X-ray examination: larynx, 156; œsophagus, 176, 181, 185; sinuses, 87
X-ray therapy, 48, 50, 123
Xylocaine, 88

Zeiss operating microscope, 235, 250

NURSING BOOKS

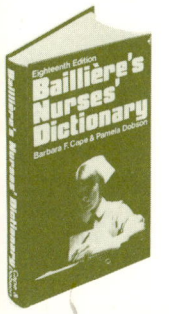

BAILLIÈRE'S NURSES' DICTIONARY
By Barbara F. Cape S.R.N., S.C.M., D.N. (Lond.)
and Pamela Dobson S.R.N., S.C.M., R.N.T.

The new 18th edition of this famous dictionary has been completely reset and updated in a new format. It contains hundreds of new definitions, radically revised appendices and new illustrations – an informative, pocket-sized dictionary for student and trained nurse alike.

18th ed   512 pages   8 plates   70p

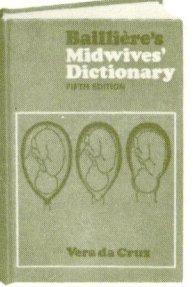

BAILLIÈRE'S MIDWIVES' DICTIONARY
By Vera Da Cruz S.R.N., S.C.M., M.T.D.

The ideal pocket-sized dictionary for midwives and obstetric nurses. "A little mine of invaluable information . . . it really does contain the exact definition wanted in a hurry."

Midwives' Chronicle 1969

5th ed   396 pages   140 illus   55p

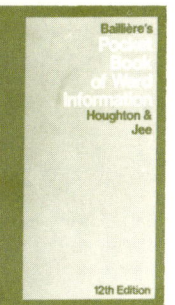

BAILLIÈRE'S POCKET BOOK OF WARD INFORMATION
By Marjorie Houghton O.B.E., S.R.N., S.C.M., D.N.
and Ann Jee S.R.N., Part 1 C.M.B., R.N.T.

Fully revised and brought up-to-date, this book contains a multitude of useful information likely to be needed by nurses in their day to day work and of particular help to nurses in training.

12th ed   192 pages   6 illus   55p

BAILLIÈRE TINDALL   7 & 8 Henrietta Street
London WC2E 8QE

REFERENCE AND SPECIALIST TEXTS

VENEREAL DISEASES: TREATMENT AND NURSING
By H. Elliott S.R.N. and K. Ryz S.R.N., R.M.N., M.I.H.E.

Knowledge of the sexually transmitted diseases is now an important part of nurse training and this new book provides essential information on this subject. It covers the infection, diagnosis and treatment of syphilis, gonorrhoea, the nonspecific genital infections and other associated conditions. The authors write sympathetically about the situations the nurse will encounter, and their experience and understanding provide much valuable insight for the reader.
200 pages   16 illus   1 colour plate   £1.80

PATIENT CARE: CARDIOVASCULAR DISORDERS
By Pat M. Ashworth S.R.N., S.C.M., and Harry Rose S.R.N., R.F.N., R.N.T., B.T.A.

This new textbook is designed for nurses who have completed some of their preliminary nursing studies and are ready to deepen their knowledge of the more specialized aspects of patient care. The authors have written a stimulating and very informative text which will be of value to both student and trained nurses.
240 pages   68 illus   £2.80

NURSES' GUIDE TO CARDIAC MONITORING
By Peter Hubner M.B., B.S., M.R.C.P.

"This small book treats the whole subject of ECG monitoring in a very practical way, with clear examples of the traces as observed on the monitor . . . The value of this book is that it is short, concise and practical in its approach . . ." *Nursing Times 1971*
66 pages   35 illus   £1.00

MAYES' MIDWIFERY: A TEXTBOOK FOR MIDWIVES
By Rosemary E. Bailey S.R.N., S.C.M., M.T.D., R.N.T., D.N.

This book has long been accepted as one of the classic textbooks for the midwife, and its clarity and completeness have been particularly welcomed by those studying for the examination of the Central Midwives Board. In this new eighth edition the text has been extensively rewritten and revised to take account of recent developments in obstetrics.
8th ed   530 pages   186 illus   £2.50

BAILLIÈRE TINDALL   7 & 8 Henrietta Street
London WC2E 8QE

DO-IT-YOURSELF REVISION FOR NURSES   BOOKS 1, 2, 3, 4, 5 & 6

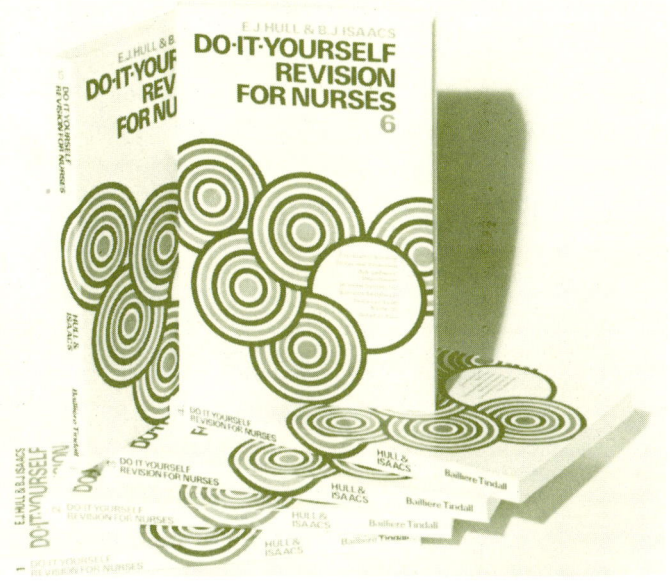

These books provide an entirely new concept which gives the nurse a systematic and interesting method of revision. Together they are planned to provide a comprehensive framework for revision for the 1969 syllabus of the General Nursing Council and developments made since to it. Each book of this unique set enables the nurse to study a particular subject, answer questions selected from recent State Final examinations and mark her replies against model answers provided. Tutors will also be interested in the set answers of experienced examiners. Books 1—6 each 60p

All you need
for quick · simple · easy 'exam' revision

BAILLIÈRE TINDALL 7 & 8 Henrietta Street
London WC2E 8QE

THE NURSES

The Nurses' Aids Series is planned to meet the needs of the student nurse during training, and later in qualifying for another part of the Register, by providing a set of textbooks covering most of the subjects included in the general part of the Register, and certain specialist subjects. The pupil nurse, too, will find many of these books of particular value and help in practical bedside training.

The Series conforms to three factors of major importance to the student:

1. All the authors are nurses who know exactly what the student requires.
2. The books are regularly revised to ensure that advances and expansion in knowledge are available to the student as soon as practicable.
3. The books are well printed and easy to read, comprehensively illustrated, compact and priced within the reach of all students.

Thus this famous Series, which covers all aspects of nursing studies—scientific, theoretical and practical—contributes significantly to nurse training in this country and abroad.

ANATOMY AND PHYSIOLOGY FOR NURSES
by K. F. Armstrong, S.R.N., S.C.M., D.N. & S. M. Jackson, S.R.N., S.C.M., B.T.A., R.N.T.
8th ed   hard £1.50   limp £1.00

ANAESTHETICS FOR NURSES
by J. Hobkirk, S.R.N.
1st ed   limp £1.00

ARITHMETIC IN NURSING
by W. C. Fream, S.R.N., B.T.A. Cert. & R. P. Davies, R.M.N., S.R.N., R.N.T., A.H.A.
4th ed   hard £1.50   limp £1.00

EAR, NOSE AND THROAT NURSING
by S. Marshall, S.R.N., S.C.M., D.N. & Z. Oxlade, S.R.N., R.N.T.
5th ed   hard £1.50   limp £1.00

MEDICAL NURSING
by M. Houghton, O.B.E., S.C.M., D.N., & C. M. Chapman, B.Sc.(Soc.), S.R.N., S.C.M., R.N.T.
8th ed   hard £1.40   limp £1.00

MICROBIOLOGY FOR NURSES
by E. J. Bocock. Revised by M. J. Parker, S.R.N.
4th ed   hard £1.40   limp £1.00

OBSTETRIC AND GYNAECOLOGICAL NURSING
by R. E. Bailey, S.R.N., S.C.M., M.T.D., R.N.T., D.N.
1st ed   hard £1.40   limp £1.00

ORTHOPAEDICS FOR NURSES
by W. Talog Davies. Revised by E. M. Stone, Hon. M.A., S.R.N., S.C.M., R.N.T.
4th ed   hard £1.40   limp £1.00

7 & 8 Henrietta Street   **BAILLIÈ**

New editions may have been published since this list was printed; pric

AIDS SERIES

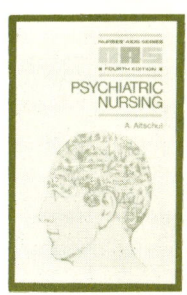

PAEDIATRIC NURSING
by M. A. Duncombe, S.R.N.,
R.S.C.N., S.C.M., & B. Weller,
S.R.N., R.S.C.N., R.N.T.
4th ed   hard £1.80   limp £1.10

**PERSONAL AND
COMMUNITY HEALTH**
by W. Huntly, S.R.N., S.C.M.,
D.N.
2nd ed   hard £1.00   limp 75p

PHARMACOLOGY FOR NURSES
by Rosemary E. Bailey, S.R.N.,
S.T.D., D.N.
3rd ed   hard £1.40   limp £1.00

PRACTICAL NURSING
revised by M. Clarke, B.Sc.,
S.R.N., R.N.T.
11th ed   hard £1.40   limp £1.00

PRACTICAL PROCEDURES
by M. Houghton, O.B.E., S.R.N.,
S.C.M., D.N., & J. E. Parnell,
S.R.N., S.C.M., R.N.T.
1st ed   limp 80p

PSYCHIATRIC NURSING
by A. Altschul, B.A., S.R.N., R.M.N.
4th ed   hard £1.50   limp £1.00

PSYCHOLOGY FOR NURSES
A. by Altschul. B.A., S.R.N., R.M.N.
3rd ed   limp £1.00

SURGICAL NURSING
by E. J. Fish, S.R.N., O.N.C.,
R.C.N.T., R.N.T.
**9th ed   382 pp   67 illus
hard £2.00   limp £1.20**

THEATRE TECHNIQUE
by M. Houghton, O.B.E.,
S.R.N., S.C.M., D.N., &
J. Hudd, S.R.N.
4th ed   limp £1.00

**TROPICAL HYGIENE
AND NURSING**
by Wm. C. Fream, S.R.N.,
B.T.A.Cert., S.T.D.
5th ed   limp 90p

TINDALL   London WC2E 8QE

details do not necessarily refer to current editions.   Each book 7" × 4½"

STANDARD TEXTBOOKS

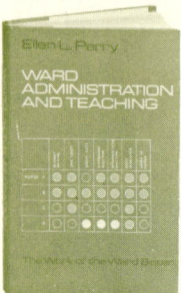

WARD ADMINISTRATION & TEACHING
By Ellen L. Perry

"This is a book which has long been needed. Every trained nurse could learn something from it. While ward sisters put into practice the ideals and ideas outlined, we need have no fears for 'patient care' in our hospitals nor for the practical training of the nurse." *Nursing Mirror*

304 pages   **11 illus**   **£2.00**

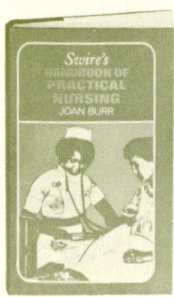

SWIRE'S HANDBOOK OF PRACTICAL NURSING
Revised by Joan Burr R.M.N., S.R.N.

Changes in the syllabus of training have necessitated a major revision for this edition and Miss Burr has taken the opportunity to make many changes of approach to stress the human angle and to enable the nurse to appreciate her surroundings in the hospital and in the community. Care has been taken to cover the syllabus fully, and the use of simple language and illustrated examples ensure the maintained interest of the pupil.

6th ed   **308 pages**   **57 illus**   **£1.10**

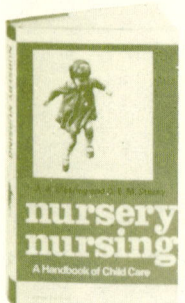

NURSERY NURSING—
A HANDBOOK FOR NURSERY NURSES
By A. B. Meering S.R.N., S.C.M.
and G. Stacey S.R.N.

"This book is written in a clear and simple style emphasizing the relationship between the emotional, intellectual and physical growth during infancy and childhood . . . a valuable reference book for all nurses interested in nursery work . . ." *The Lamp*

5th ed   **414 pages**   **75 illus**   **£2.50**

BAILLIÈRE TINDALL   7 & 8 Henrietta Street
London WC2E 8QE